Spiritual Care and Transcultural Care Research

Note

Health care practice and knowledge are constantly changing and developing as new research and treatments, changes in procedures, drugs and equipment become available.

The author and publishers have, as far as is possible, taken care to confirm that the information complies with the latest standards of practice and legislation.

Spiritual Care and Transcultural Care Research

Aru Narayanasamy

Associate Professor, School of Nursing, University of Nottingham, Queen's Medical Centre, Nottingham

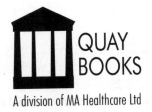

QUAY
BOOKS

A division of MA Healthcare Ltd

Quay Books Division, MA Healthcare Ltd, St Jude's Church, Dulwich Road, London SE24 0PB

British Library Cataloguing-in-Publication Data
A catalogue record is available for this book

© MA Healthcare Limited 2006

ISBN 1 85642 298 4

Printed by Gutenberg Press Limited, Gudja Road, Tarxien PLA19, Malta

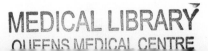

Foreword

Barbara Parfitt

It is difficult to deny even in this age of science and technology the existence of a dimension of life that goes beyond the purely physical. Whether or not we are religious, in each of us there is a desire to understand what meaning and purpose our lives have. When we are young and physically fit this search for meaning and purpose can be suppressed and ignored as we engage with the physical aspects of our lives. When, however, we are frail, sick or suffering, either emotionally or physically, it is then we realise that the innate desire of human kind is to understand our origins and to explain the purpose of our existence. How we express this search often reflects the culture from which we have learned our core values and beliefs. But regardless of our different cultures and religious expressions of faith, the urge to understand our spiritual core remains the same.

Nurses and other health professionals are faced with patients and clients who need their support and care, which means that an acknowledgement of the spiritual dimension of life is essential if we hope to meet the needs of our patients in a holistic way. Holism implies the embracing of a model of care that takes account of all aspects of human existence, including the spiritual and cultural. Suffering is part of the human state and to pretend that we all have the right to be without any suffering is to fail to learn how to provide care to those in spiritual distress. Within the Western model of health care delivery, wherever it is delivered in the world, the provision of spiritual care is often sadly lacking. Not only do we not understand our own spiritual needs, we also fail to understand those of our patients or clients and so are unable to fully care for them. As Dr Narayanasamy says 'we leave our distressed patients to struggle on their own' (p. 2).

It has been said that those who do not have either a personal faith or a set of beliefs and values that acknowledge the spiritual dimension cannot in turn give care to those who are in spiritual distress. This reasoning could suggest that we cannot care for anyone unless we personally have suffered the same condition, which cannot be the case. The theological, philosophical and social scientific roots as presented in this text provide the foundation not only for an analysis of the coping mechanisms used by patients to meet their spiritual needs but also a model of practice for nurses and health care providers regardless of their own beliefs. This model has been rigorously underpinned by research evidence and provides an evidence base for practice in providing spiritual care.

This book will provide a much needed resource for those who know that the provision of holistic care includes the spiritual and cultural dimension. It will provide a challenge and inspiration to its readers.

Barbara Parfitt PhD, RGN, RM, FNP
Dean and Professor of Nursing
Glasgow Caledonian University
Glasgow
G66 4RW

Preface

Spirituality and culture feature as the central themes of this book. It represents some 15 years of research into the spiritual and cultural dimensions of care, and reflections of many more years of professional and life experiences. There is abundant evidence in the form of published literature, ranging from peer-reviewed papers to books, to suggest the importance of a holistic approach to care in order to meet the needs of patients and clients with regard to the body, mind, spirit and culture. All of these dimensions are integral to an individual's personhood and sense of being. Increasingly, health and social care practitioners are called upon or challenged to respond to the holistic needs of their patients/clients, which may be overt or covert at times. This means that a holistic approach (care of the body, mind and spirit) is paramount in the context of health and social care. The harmonious balance between the body, mind and spirit is central to the very existence of a person. Emerging empirical evidence suggests that a responsive and sensitive approach to the holistic needs of patients/clients may lead to healing and holistic restoration of the person affected by ill health or life crises.

All the studies reported in this book emerged from the Bearings Project: The Bearings of Empirical Studies of Spirituality and Culture on Nurse Education, and have been published in various professional journals. When the findings of studies are published as individual papers in disparate journals, there is sometimes a danger that it becomes difficult to capture the coherent and developmental nature of the research programme, such as the studies forming the central themes; that is, the spiritual and cultural dimensions of care in this book. As the project leader of the Bearings Project, it has been my privilege to bring together a collection of studies to share with others who are contemplating upon embarking on an empirical pursuit of a similar nature as health/social care practitioners and students or as readers interested in the fields of spirituality and culture.

The book therefore charts a systematic and sustained approach to research into this important area of humanity and includes five studies on spirituality and culture in the context of nurse education and health care. The early sections of the book (Chapters 1–3) provide conceptual clarification on the topics of spirituality and culture in health care. Subsequent chapters comprise reports of findings from the research into spiritual and cultural care conducted as part of the Bearings Project. These chapters have been presented in a sequence that demonstrates the coherent and developmental nature of my work, where one enquiry has led to another. It is hoped that readers will be able to derive insights into the various narratives that patients, nurses/health carers and students provided about their lived experience of respectively receiving and giving spiritual and cultural care.

A helping hand with attributes of spiritual and cultural care considerations is an extension of our love and compassion for people who find themselves as strangers in health care. In a way, when we talk about spiritual and cultural care, we are inevitably putting into action the notion 'Loving the stranger', requiring health and social care. I have made every attempt to ensure the accuracy of the material of this book. I have also exercised a great sense of sensitivity and ethically considerations in my endeavour to contribute to the enhancement of quality of life for those who need our attention, who are often in suffering and distress beyond their control. I extend my sincere apologies for any omissions or errors.

Finally, this book also reflects the trend in the conceptual and theoretical understanding of spirituality and culture in the context of health care. It is hoped that readers will share with me the conceptual, empirical, and reflective literature that abounds in this book.

Aru Narayanasamy
April 2006

Acknowledgements

I would like to express my thanks to Mr David Henderson, former Chief Executive of Trinity Care, part of Southern Cross Health Care Group, for helping me to secure funding for the Bearings Project and for his continued support, and I would like to thank Dr Mervyn Suffield, former Director of Care, Trinity Care, for his support at the early stages of this project. I am also grateful to all the participants of my studies, to both the external and internal reviewers of my published works and to Professor Bob Gates, Professor John Swinton and Ethelerene White for their contribution to the chapters in this book. I thank Helen Scott, former editor of the *British Journal of Nursing*, for giving permission to publish respective *BJN* articles as book chapters. Finally, my thanks go to my wife Mani, my son Gavin and my daughter Melanie for their unfailing love, affection and support for me throughout my studies and the writing of this book.

Contents

Contributors

Professor Bob Gates, Head of Learning Disabilities, Thames Valley University

Professor John Swinton, Professor of Theology and Practical Pastoral Care, University of Aberdeen

Dr Aru Narayanasamy, Associate Professor/Director of Staff Development, Faculty of Medicine and Health Sciences, School of Nursing, University of Nottingham.

Mrs Mani Narayanasamy, Registered Nurse (Health Promotion), Nottingham.

Mrs Ethelrene White, Health Lecturer, Faculty of Medicine and Health Sciences, School of Nursing, University of Nottingham.

Disclaimer

Every attempt has been made to ensure the accuracy of the material present in this book. Issues arising from spiritual and cultural data and other perspectives have been treated with due care and sensitivity. This book has been written to reflect my commitment to promoting holistic care and enhancing quality of life for people facing spiritual and cultural distress whilst their lives are shattered by health crisis or suffering. Much of the book is about being a sensitive companion to the broken person to heal in body, mind and spirit. Apologies are extended to readers in advance if there has been any omission or mistake. This will be rectified at the earliest opportunity.

CHAPTER I

Introduction

Scientific medicine and medical technologies make a significant impact upon the lives of those affected by health problems as well as those seeking perfection in body for aesthetic reasons. Whilst many recoveries from illness and trauma are due to advances in medical, nursing and health care, some people do not recover. On the other hand, some recover in spite of the limitations of medical care. I believe that there is something within or outside a person that helps with the recovery. The research presented in this book is based on my conviction that spirituality and culture are integral to the wellbeing of an individual. I have come across several narratives, as told by patients and carers, as well as my lived experiences as a health carer, witnessing miraculous recoveries or healing. I came across these testimonies as a professional caring for those afflicted by illness or trauma as they struggle with their brokenness as a person and their journey in suffering to be restored as a physical, psychological and spiritual being.

Increasingly, I began to realise the power and limitations of scientific medicine in its attempts to restore the affected person to full health. When medicine failed, something else took over and made healing possible. Sometimes, a seemingly unscientific endeavour, like the promise of a visit from a relative travelling a long distance, gave the patient the will to live long enough until the visit took place. I remember Patrick (not his real name) dying soon after his sister visited him from Australia. I also realised that at times nothing works for patients and I felt helpless as I and other health professionals were powerless to do anything but keep them as comfortable as possible. I became increasingly committed to the notion of holistic care, that is, care of the person's body, mind and spirit in their suffering as they make the journey towards recovery, which could be slow, steady or rapid, or at times impossible. I believe in the power of spiritual and cultural care. Much of the focus of this book is about these two important dimensions of humanity. Helping the sick or the traumatised to regain their individuality as a wholesome person is a privilege. I hold this privilege dearly and treasure the memories of the person making progress through holistic care, that is, the care that touches the very core of the person, the spirit. It is a satisfying experience. Evidence from my research and others supports the idea that nurses themselves derive much satisfaction from providing spiritual care to their patients (Narayanasamy *et al.*, 2004; O'Brien, 2003).

Spirituality is a term that keeps cropping up throughout health care and its literature. What is obvious is that spirituality contains a multiplicity of meanings. Sometimes the plasticity and ambiguity of the concept allows for deep misunderstandings as well as misuse. For the purpose of this book, spirituality is defined as 'the essence of our being and it gives meaning and purpose to our existence' (Narayanasamy, 2004).

Burkhardt and Nagai-Jacobson (2002, p. 94) elaborate the concept of spirituality: 'Spirituality permeates life; shapes our life journey; and is vital to the process of discovering purpose, meaning, and inner strength'. Various definitions, descriptions and disputes about spirituality and culture are explored throughout this book. I heard once someone saying, 'It takes an enormous amount of grace to negotiate through the minefield of disagreement'. Healthy debates are necessary in exploring disputes about concepts, caring practices and related issues, but ultimately the wellbeing of our patients is what matters, and whatever we do should make a difference to their lives. I believe that health professionals can reach out to the patient's spirituality by the 5 'C's – Caring, Compassion, Connection, Communication and Commitment – when they face distress, illness, trauma or death. These are the central themes of this book. Even if we feel incapable of addressing patient's spiritual and cultural needs through lack of knowledge and competence or our own human vulnerability in trying and demanding circumstances, we can still reach out to our patients by 'presencing' – simply being there – when a patient needs a companion in their suffering and brokenness. Through caring and compassionate presencing we can transcend cultural barriers. We can connect and communicate with our patients.

Connection goes in hand with simplicity in our approach to spiritual and cultural needs. There is something elegant about simplicity and much of this book is about translating abstract theories of spirituality and culture, and the lived experiences of people, into applied realities in making the differences to patients' lives in their struggle to regain their identity as a whole (holistic) person – a person with a culture and history, a person with body, mind and spirit.

This book incorporates the scholarly contribution to the field of nursing made by the spiritual and cultural care research programme known as the Bearings Project. The intention of this chapter is to provide an overview of the project to enable the reader to make sense of a body of work resulting from personal, professional and intellectual development and commitment to spiritual and cultural care research. The commitment to the research programme came about as a result of the concern within nursing that the provision of spiritual care for patients is inadequate (Swinton, 2001; Greenstreet, 1999; Oldnall, 1995, 1996; McGilloway and Myco, 1983; Soeken and Carson, 1987; Millison, 1988).

The nurse's role is described as an 'inspiriting' one, providing a sense of identity, worth, hope and purpose in existence (Jourard, 1974; Jacik, 1986). By implication the inspiriting role can be perceived as giving spiritual care; however, if the provision of spiritual care is inadequate, this means leaving the distressed patient to cope on their own in their struggle with spirituality. Consequently, the patient becomes distressed spiritually and may have to endure further suffering, often compounded by problems of pain, low self-esteem, feelings of isolation, powerless, hopelessness and anger. There is evidence to suggest that learning opportunities in nursing are often limited to physical needs, and that information about spirituality is neglected (Greenstreet, 1999; Piles, 1986; Highfield and Cason, 1983). Emerging research calls for educational strategies to be in place to prepare nurses for spiritual caregiving (Greenstreet, 1999). Added to this is anecdotal evidence of similar concern from many health care professionals that I have interacted with over the years. Furthermore, I have witnessed many incidents of spontaneous recoveries in which medicine had no or little role in these miracles. After a prolonged period of reflection and search I came to the conclusion that spirituality and faith must play an important role in these recoveries and healing. I will recount some of these experiences next.

In my early clinical years, I witnessed on a medical ward a patient known as Fred (not his real name), considered to be at the end of life, making a spontaneous recovery. The medical profession was unable to offer an explanation for why and how this spontaneous recovery happened. Doctors instructed the nurses to stop making any heroic attempt to resuscitate Fred if he went into cardiac arrest. We were asked to keep the patient comfortable and do nothing more. Before I left for my long-awaited two-day break, I whispered to this debilitated, comatose patient 'Goodbye', with the sure knowledge that Fred would be dead by my next shift. When I returned to resume my next shift following the short break, I was horrified initially, but delighted at the same time, to see Fred dashing around the ward and being helpful to other patients. I could not believe my eyes, as Fred was at the brink of death before I went away, but was now full of life – nothing would stop him. It was a miracle that remains indelible in my mind to date. At the time doctors could not explain and were dismissive of it as a rare instance of spontaneous recovery. This incident raised many questions, and I can only put it down to something beyond us that was responsible for his recovery and gave him a chance to live again. Later I gathered from his visitors that his relatives and close friends locally and as far afield as Australia had held a prayer vigil for him. I am certain that it was spirituality rather than medicine that was responsible for Fred's spontaneous recovery. He was discharged within days.

Another incident reminds me of the role of faith in healing.

Tom, a devout Christian, fell and fractured his femur. He was X-rayed at the hospital and it revealed more than the fracture to his femur: there were cancerous metastases to his bone. Tom was subjected to further tests and it confirmed that he had primaries in his lungs and these had spread to his bones and other parts of his body. The specialist told Tom that apart from the treatment of his fracture, there was nothing he could do for him. I saw Tom, cheerful as ever, three years later, walking with his wife. In my experience, many people who had similar conditions to Tom normally died within months. I am sure it was his faith that healed and sustained him.

Rout (1990), in his book on miracles of healing, provides several accounts of patients who have defied serious forms of cancer and have lived long enough to tell tales of their recovery. In some cases the primary cancerous growths had shrunk or disappeared completely. Rout attributes such miraculous recoveries to the power of spirituality as the major contributory factor when medicine had failed. In some cases patients had ignored aggressive treatment regimes by turning to spiritual sources to regain strength and healing. According to Rout, medical practitioners who dealt with these patients attributed such miracles to spontaneous remissions and failed to give weight to interventions beyond their control. Clearly Rout's work illustrates that where medicine fails, spirituality takes over.

Spirituality and health care

Scholars indicate the possibility of the universality of spirituality and its clinical significance. The classic work of Otto (1950), James (1983), Hardy (1987) and Smart (1996) presents evidence to suggest the universality and enduring nature of spirituality as a significant human experience. Other contemporary research, including the empirical work of Hay and Nye (1998) and Hay and Hunt (2002) has indicated that the general population has a strong and indeed growing sense of spiritual awareness. Others, including Davies (1994), map a continuing rise of spiritual awareness in western societies. The neurological work of Newberg *et al.* (2002), using sophisticated scanning techniques, presents scientific evidence supporting the universal presence of spirituality in human beings which, they argue, exists for evolutionary purposes. Furthermore, there is evidence that patients in the USA and UK actually desire and expect their spiritual dimensions to be cared for (Beeforth, 1997; Fitchett *et al.*, 1997; Charters, 1999). Whilst church attendance is in decline in the UK, there is an upsurge in the so-called 'New Age spirituality' (Utley, 2003). A growing body of literature also suggests that spirituality has significant health benefits, and the incorporation of this dimension into clinical practice can lead to improved forms of care (Dossey, 1993; Larson *et al.*, 1997; Koenig *et al.*, 2000; Swinton and Narayanasamy, 2002; Baldacchino, 2003). The implications of this literature are that caregivers need to recognise that sensitivity to a patient's spiritual needs is critical if they are to provide truly 'holistic care', that is, attention to the body, mind and spirit.

Spirituality and culture

As soon as I embarked on the research I became increasingly aware of the connection between spirituality and culture, and its significance for health care. On further reflection I also became aware that the cultural dimension was frequently overlooked, in so far as it was also inadequately addressed within the caring context (Ahmad, 1993; Fernando, 1995; Gerrish *et al.*, 1996; Le Var, 1998; Gerrish and Papadopoulos, 1999; Chady, 2001; Serrant Green, 2001). Inadequate educational, research and practice provisions have been blamed in the past for the lack of pace in the development of transcultural nursing. However, since the early 1990s a body of evidence on transcultural nursing has begun to emerge within the UK, most notably the work of Gerrish (1997), Papadapolous *et al.* (2004) and McGee (1992) to guide cultural care.

Furthermore, as the subject theme leader for the spiritual and cultural dimensions of care, I became increasingly aware of the slow development of theory and the lack of models of spiritual and cultural care in health care. In the light of this I began to investigate and disseminate the findings of my work on the spiritual and cultural dimensions of care. At an early stage of the research I received substantial financial sponsorship (£30,000) from Trinity Care plc and £1000 from the ENB. These sponsorships helped to fund subsequent research.

Collaboration in terms of research, publication and interactions between fellow professionals and myself in the setting of a research-led university has been an important vehicle for my endeavour within spiritual and cultural care research. Professional colleagues and the Bearings Project Team (Narayanasamy *et al.*, 2004) have acted as a community of critical friends who have ensured that knowledge creation and innovations retained their integrity within the long process of enquiry. They acted as 'reality checkers' for my intellectual enquiry and helped to counteract the negative impact of values and bias that researchers bring to the enquiry process as a consequence of cultural, spiritual, psychological and philosophical influences.

Aims of the research programme

The aims of the research programme were derived from my experience as a scholar/practitioner in health care. They are:

1. To establish and develop empirical studies of spirituality and culture.
2. To generate knowledge through personal and collaborative scholarship.
3. To disseminate research findings on the significance of spiritual and cultural care in order that they can inform nurse education and nursing practice.

Each of these aims has been addressed through research and publications as part of the Bearings Project, with related objectives, over the past 10 years.

Description of the research programme

This book embraces two interrelated fields of work. The first one – spiritual dimensions of care education and practice (Chapters 2, 4, 5 and 6) – offers a range of theoretical and empirical data as well as a model for spirituality and spiritual care education, while the second field – cultural dimensions of care (Chapters 3 and 8) – provides theoretical perspectives and a model for cultural care.

The various chapters of this book reflect a mix of empirical and conceptual work, with some contribution to theoretical knowledge and development of models of education and practice. Chapters 4, 5, 6 and 8 represent original empirical research and Chapters 2 and 8 develop conceptual models or theoretical ideas. The contents of these chapters together represent a body of interrelated knowledge whilst acknowledging the distinctness of each field.

The data and theoretical models are from a range of sources. These include personal scholarship, specific research collaborations with other scholars (Professor John Swinton; Professor Bob Gates and Ahmed Andrews), and a funded research project at the University of Nottingham. This Bearings Project represents the bearings of empirical studies of spirituality and culture on nurse education.

Some methodological issues

The holistic and multi-perspective nature of spirituality and culture requires a multidisciplinary approach and a flexibility of methodology, so a range of research techniques was used. These include descriptive statistical analysis, content and thematic analyses (Chapters 4, 5, 6 and 7); interviews and phenomenological protocol analysis (Chapter 4); critical incident techniques with reflective interviews (Chapters 5 and 6); and action research (Chapter 8). My academic background in research methods in applied social sciences and education, health care, and research training as part of a funded research project (Day *et al.*, 1998) influenced my selection of research methods. My experience as an action researcher in applied social sciences laid the foundation for managing research projects. Much of the project used action research, which facilitated a collaborative and participatory process in which researchers and participants work together by actioning, evaluating and modifying practices continuously to bring about new knowledge and practice (Altrichter *et al.*, 1993; Rolfe *et al.*, 2001; Waterman *et al.*, 2001).

Chapter summaries

Chapters 2 and 3 respectively comprise conceptual literature on spirituality and culture. A holistic understanding of spirituality rooted in theology, philosophy and the social sciences is developed in Chapter 2. It raises some pertinent points surrounding the notions of spirituality and religion and attempts to offer a working definition of spirituality in the light of contemporary thinking. Likewise, in Chapter 3 transcultural perspectives are examined in the context of current literature in the field. In so doing, the key features of transcultural nursing are explored and commented upon in terms of the following: definitions, racism, ethnocentrism, culture, diversity, transcultural health care practice, legislation and reports, transcultural health care nurse education and models of practice. There is promising evidence from emerging literature that innovations are taking place in promoting transcultural care practice and education, but the pace remains somewhat slow.

Chapter 4 illuminates the findings of a qualitative study of spiritual coping mechanisms in chronically ill patients. In the UK little is known about the lived experience of spiritual coping mechanisms in chronic illness due to a lack of empirical evidence. In response to the gap in the literature and research related to spiritual coping mechanisms in chronically ill patients, this chapter contributes to empirical knowledge as a unique study in the UK. The findings highlight the lived experience of spiritual mechanisms where connectedness (Sherwood, 2000; Reed, 1992; Granstrom, 1985) with God through prayer and connectedness with others appear to be significant part of the healing process in chronic illness.

The limitation of this study is that it offers only a partial picture with regard to spiritual coping mechanisms due to the fact that the majority of participants were adherents of religious faiths. Further research is needed in a variety of clinical settings to map out the specific nature of spiritual coping mechanisms in both believers and non-believers. However, the chapter opens up this area of research by offering an insight into the spiritual coping mechanisms of chronically ill patients. The implications of this study are that patients may benefit from nursing interventions which are sensitive, supportive and responsive to their spiritual needs.

Chapters 5 and 6 contain findings of critical incident studies of nurses' responses to the spiritual needs of their patients. Both chapters, based on collaborative work, are the first of their kind to offer scope for theory and practice development in nursing using this approach. In particular, these chapters illuminate professional commitment to person-centredness, engagement, interpersonal attributes, involvement and sensitivity to spiritual needs as features of ideal spiritual care practice (O'Brien, 2003; Tanyi, 2002; Sanders, 2002). However, the research study in Chapter 5 was limited in that the sample did not include learning disabilities nurses, so the study in Chapter 6 was developed to show how nurses caring for people with learning disabilities respond to clients' spiritual needs. Professor Bob Gates and Professor John Swinton, as co-authors and research collaborators, shared valuable insights into learning disabilities and the literature when developing Chapter 6.

Chapters 7 and 8 refer to a conceptual model and empirical data with regard to transcultural health care. These chapters offer a model for transcultural mental nursing. It emerged in my work that spirituality and culture are integral to many people's lives. In particular, an apparent lack of transcultural perspectives on mental health care practice began to emerge. The ACCESS model is a unique and innovative development and is grounded in the theoretical perspectives derived from transcultural practice-based literature (Papadopoulos *et al.*, 2004; Peberdy, 1997; Leininger, 1997; Ahuarangi, 1996; Gerrish *et al.*, 1996; Goode, 1993; Sherer, 1993; Dobson, 1991) and empirical data derived from an unpublished survey study (Narayanasamy, 1998b) that I carried out, in which participants ($n = 36$) who had educational input through this model suggest that 85% of respondents found it highly useful for transcultural mental health care practice.

The theoretical perspectives on cultural dimensions of care influence scholarly exposition on the subject of transcultural mental health care (Clegg, 2003; Chady, 2001; Eisenbruch, 2001; Holland and Hogg, 2001). Chady developed a perspective on the National Service Framework for Mental Health that is based on my work. The ACCESS model as described in Chapter 7 formed the basis for the transcultural health care education offered at the University of Nottingham. The limitation of the study given in these chapters is that they are based on a small sample and it is therefore difficult to generalise the application of the ACCESS model. However, according to Chady (2001, p. 988), 'the ACCESS model in its entirety creates a demand for training and supervision structures involving the experiences of culture specific voluntary providers as well as the influence of expert panels'. Likewise, Eisenbruch (2001, p. 11) suggests that the ACCESS model advances 'an alternative to this ethnocentric style of nurse education in cultural competence'. An evaluation study of this model is reported in Chapter 8.

Chapter 7 provides empirical data from a study of Registered Nurses ($n = 126$) to suggest that a majority of respondents claimed that they feel that patients' cultural needs should be given consideration. Cultural aspects of care seem to be a feature of the overall picture of nursing within multicultural context of health care. Many participants claimed that they responded to the cultural needs of patients recently. A number of them felt that patients' cultural needs are adequately met, but these needs were perceived to be religious practices, diets, communication, dying, prayer and culture. Furthermore, a significant number of respondents suggested that they would like further education in meeting the cultural needs of their patients.

Chapter 8 provides empirical data from a study in which participants ($n = 166$) who received transcultural health care education completed questionnaires with statements about the usefulness of this model. The findings suggest that 90% ($n = 149$) of participants found the model to be very useful. In spite of its limitations with respect to the lack of user perspectives on the usefulness of the model, this chapter is valuable for the theory and practice of transcultural nursing and education. According to Chady (2001), Eisenbruch (2001), Holland and Hogg (2001) and Stanley (2000) the ACCESS model offers a useful framework for nurses implementing transcultural care practice. This was confirmed when I presented a paper on this model at a national conference held in April 2002 at De Montfort University (Narayanasamy, 2002). 'ACCESS' as an acronym enables nurses to be consciously aware of its central features when carrying out nursing care of minority ethnic patients. In summary, the ACCESS model is a unique development within nursing and there is empirical evidence from this publication to support its usefulness as a transcultural nursing framework.

The main limitation of this study is that the relationship between nurses' experience and education could have been explored to establish the link between attitudes shaped by education and transcultural care practice. However, in spite of these limitations this study contributes to empirical understanding in nursing education and practice by offering insights into how nurses meet the cultural needs of their clients. This publication and the ACCESS model proposed in Chapters 7 and 8 guide curriculum developers in devising appropriate educational programmes for improving transcultural health care practices for nursing and nurse education.

Previous research has shown that most nurses want or need information about spirituality (Harrison, 1993; Narayanasamy, 1993; Oldnall, 1995; Ross, 1997; Hawley, 2002; Sanders, 2002; Tanyi, 2002). Chapter 9 provides a synthesis of my conceptual and empirical work to illustrate how my publications have become key collections on the theory and practice of spiritual and cultural dimensions of care for nurse education (Hawley, 2002). In line with the theoretical perspectives of other scholars (Baldacchino, 2003; Aldridge, 2000; Swinton, 2002; McSherry, 2000; Henley and Schott, 1999), the significance of spiritual and cultural pluralism in contemporary Britain is highlighted. However, there are limitations in my work. It is acknowledged that no research is perfect in that it leaves scope for criticisms of oversights or omissions with regard to the theoretical perspectives. Furthermore, in its attempts to reconcile the theoretical and practice nature of spiritual and cultural care, there is the danger that some aspects of the discourse in the book are trivialised or marginalised. However, it is hoped that spiritual and transcultural care practice is being informed by this research. Hawley (2002, p. 118) adds: '...it increases the availability of spiritual writings for those involved in nursing education today, be that student or teachers'. Likewise, Eisenbruch (2001) notes that the ACCESS model is a practical alternative to the ethnocentric style of nurse education in competence. Finally, I believe that if the various themes of this book are taken together, they provide a body of evidence which is central to education and practice.

References

Ahmad, W. I. U. (1993) *Race and Health in Contemporary Britain*. Open University Press, Buckingham.

Ahuarangi, K. C. (1996) Creating a safe cultural space. *Kai Tiaki: Nursing New Zealand*, November, 13–15.

Aldridge, D. (2000) *Spirituality, Healing and Medicine*. Jessica Kingsley, London.

Altrichter, H., Posch, P. and Somekh, B. (1993) *Teachers Investigate their Work: An Introduction to the Methods of Action Research*. Routledge, London.

Aveyard, B. (1995) A question of faith. *Nursing Standard*, **9**(37), 45–6.

Baldacchino, D. (2003) *Spirituality in Illness and Care*. Price Library, Malta.

Bearings Project (2002) `http://www.nottingham.ac.uk/healthquest/staff/an-bearingsproject.html`.

Beeforth, M. (1997) *Knowing Our Own Minds*. The Mental Health Foundation, London.

Burkhardt, M. A. and Nagai-Jacobson, M. G. (2002) *Spirituality. Living our connectedness*. Delmar Thomson Learning, Australia.

Chadwick, R. (1973) Awareness and preparedness of nurses to meet spiritual needs. *The Nurses Lamp*, **22**(6), 2–3.

Chady, S. (2001) The NSF for mental health from a transcultural perspective. *British Journal of Nursing*, **10**(15), 984–90.

Charters, P. J. (1999) The religious and spiritual needs of mental health clients. *Nursing Standard*, **13**(26), 34–6.

Clegg, A. (2003) Older South Asian patient and carer perceptions of culturally sensitive care in a community hospital setting. *Journal of Clinical Nursing*, **12**, 283–90.

Curtis, M. (2000) The ghost in the machine. *Learning Disabilities Practice*, **3**(2), 11–12.

Davies, G. (1994) *Religion in Britain Since 1945*. Blackwell, Cambridge.

Day, C., Fraser, D. and Mallik, M. (1998) *The Role of the Teacher/Lecturer in Practice*. ENB, London.

Dobson, S. (1991) *Transcultural Nursing: A Contemporary Imperative*. Scutari, London.

Dossey, L. (1993) *Healing Words: the Power of Prayer and the Practice of Medicine*. Harper, San Francisco.

Eisenbruch, M. (2001) *National Review of Nursing Education: Multicultural Nursing Education*. Department of Education, Training and Youth Affairs, Commonwealth of Australia.

Fernando, S. (1995) *Mental Health in a Multiethnic Society*. Routledge, London.

Fitchett, G. (1995) Linda Krauss and the lap of God: A spiritual assessment case study. *Second Opinion*, **20**(4), 40–9.

Fitchett, G., Burton, L. A. and Sivan, A. B. (1997) The religious needs and resources of psychiatric in-patients. *Journal of Nervous and Mental Disease*, **185**(5), 320–6.

Gerrish, K. (1997) Preparation of nurses to meet the needs of an ethnically diverse society: educational implications. *Nurse Education Today*, **17**, 359–65.

Gerrish, K. and Papadopoulos, I. (1999) Transcultural competence: the challenge for nurse education. *British Journal of Nursing*, **8**(21), 1453–7.

Gerrish, K., Husband, C. and Mackenzie, J. (1996) *Nursing for a Multiethnic Society*. University Press, London.

Goode, E. E. (1993) The cultures of illness. *US News and World Report*, **114**(6), 74–6.

Granstrom, S. L. (1985) Spiritual nursing care for oncology patient. *Clinical Nursing*, **7**(1), 39–45.

Greenstreet, W. M. (1999) Teaching spirituality in nursing: a literature review. *Nurse Education Today*, **19**, 649–58.

Hardy, A. (1987) *The Spiritual Nature of Man*. Oxford University Press, Oxford.

Harrison, J. (1993) Spirituality and nursing practice. *Journal of Clinical Nursing*, **2**, 211–17.

Hay, D. and Hunt, K. (2002) *Understanding the Spirituality of People Who Don't Go to Church – The Final Report of the Adult Spirituality Spirituality Project*. University of Nottingham, Nottingham.

Hay, D. and Nye, R. (1998) *The Spirit of the Child*. HarperCollins, London.

Hawley, G. (2002) Book review: spiritual care. *Nurse Education Today*, **22**(8), 669.

Henley, A. and Schott, J. (1999) *Culture, Religion and Patient Care in a Multiethnic Society*. Age Concern, London.

Highfield, M. F. and Cason, C. (1983) Spiritual needs of patients: are they recognised? *Cancer Nursing*, June, 187–92.

Holland, K. and Hogg, C. (2001) *Cultural Awareness in Nursing and Health Care: an Introductory Text*. Arnold, London.

James, W. (1983) *The Varieties of Religious Experience*. Penguin Books, London.

Jacik, M. (1986) Personal communcation. In *Spiritual Dimensions of Nursing Practice* (ed. V. B. Carson). W. B. Saunders Company, Philadelphia.

Jourard, S. (1974) *The Transparent Self*. Van Nostrand Reinhold, New York.

Koenig, H. G., McCullough, M. E. and Larson, D. B. (2000) *Handbook of Religion and Health*. Oxford University Press, Oxford.

Larson, D. B., Swyers, J. P. and McCullough, M. (1997) *Scientific Research on Spirituality and Health: a Consensus Report*. National Institute for Healthcare Research, Rockville, Maryland.

Leininger, M. (1997) Transcultural nursing research to transcultural nursing education and practice. 40 years. *Image Journal of Nursing Scholarship*, **29**(4), 341–7.

Le Var, R. M. H. (1998) Improving educational preparation for transcultural health care. *Nurse Education Today*, **18**, 519–33.

McGee, P. (1992) *Issues in Transcultural Nursing: A Guide for Teachers of Nursing and Health*. Chapman & Hall, London.

McGilloway, O. and Myco, F. (1983) *Nursing and Spiritual Care*. Harper & Row, London.

McSherry, W. (2000) *Making Sense of Spirituality in Nursing Practice*. Churchill Livingstone, Edinburgh.

McSherry, W. (2001) Spiritual crisis? Call a nurse. In *Spirituality in Health Care Contexts* (ed. H. Orchard), pp. 107–17. Jessica Kingsley, London.

Millison, M. B. (1988) Spirituality and the caregiver, developing an under-utilised facet of care. *The American Journal of Hospice Care*, March/April, 37–44.

Narayanasamy, A. (1993) Nurses' awareness and preparedness in meeting their patients' spiritual needs. *Nurse Education Today*, **13**(4), 196–201.

Narayanasamy, A. (1998a) Religious and spiritual needs of older people. *Promoting Positive Practice in Nursing Older People*, pp. 128–50. Baillière Tindall, London.

Narayanasamy A (1998b) The ACCESS model. *Unpublished Paper*. University of Nottingham.

Narayanasamy, A. (2002) The ACCESS model: a transcultural nursing practice framework. *British Journal of Nursing*, **11**(9), 643–50.

Narayanasamy, A. (2004) The puzzle of spirituality for nursing: a guide to practical assessment. *British Journal of Nursing*, **13**(19), 1140–4.

Narayanasamy, A., Clisset, P., Annasamy, S., Edge, R., Parumal, L. and Thompson, D. (2004) A qualitative study of nurses responses to the spiritual needs of older people. *Journal of Advanced Nursing*, **48**(1), 6–16.

Newberg, A., D'Aquili, E. and Rause, V. (2002) *Why God Won't Go Away: Brain Science and the Biology of Belief*. Ballantine Books, New York.

O'Brien, M. E. (2003) *Spirituality in Nursing: Standing on Holy Ground*, 2nd edn. Jones and Barlett Publishers, Boston.

Oldnall, A. (1995) On the absence of spirituality in nursing theories and models. *Journal of Advanced Nursing*, **21**(3), 417–18.

Oldnall, A. (1996) A critical analysis of nursing: meeting the spiritual needs of patients. *Journal of Advanced Nursing*, **23**, 138–44.

Otto, R. (1950) *The Idea of the Holy* (transl. John W. Harvey). Oxford University Press, Oxford.

Papadopoulos, I., Tilki, M. and Taylor, G. (2004) *Transcultural Care: A Guide for Healthcare Professionals*, 2nd edn. Quay Books, Wiltshire.

Peberdy, A. (1997) Communicating across cultural boundaries. In: *Debates and Dilemmas in Promoting Health: A Reader* (eds. M. Siddle, L. Jones, J. Katz and A. Peberdy), pp. 99–107. Open University, Buckinghamshire.

Piles, C. (1986) Spiritual care: role of nursing education and practice: a needs survey for curriculum development. *Unpublished doctoral dissertation*. St Louis University, USA.

Reed, P. G. (1992) An emerging paradigm for the investigation of spirituality in nursing. *Research in Nursing & Health*, **15**, 349–57.

Rolfe, G., Freshwater, D. and Jasper, M. (2001) *Critical Reflection for Nurses*. Palgrave, Basingstoke.

Ross, L. (1997) *Nurses' Perceptions of Spiritual Care. Developments in Nursing and Health Care*. Avebury, Aldershot.

Rout, P. C. (1990) *Making Miracles*. Thorsons Publishing Group, Wellingborough.

Sanders, C. (2002) Challenge for spiritual care-giving in the millennium. *Contemporary Nurse*, **12**(2), 107–111.

Serrant Green, L. (2001) Transcultural nursing education: a view from within. *Nurse Education Today*, **21**(8), 670–8.

Sherwood, G. D. (2000) The power of nurse–client encounters. *Journal of Holistic Nursing*, **18**(2), 159–75.

Sherer, J. L. (1993) Crossing cultures: hospitals begins breaking down the barriers to care. *Hospitals*, **67**(10), 29–31.

Smart, N. (1996) *The Religious Experience of Mankind*, 5th edn. Prentice Hall, New Jersey.

Soeken, K. L. and Carson, V. J. (1987) Responding to the spiritual needs of the chronically ill. *Nursing Clinics of North America*, **22**(3), 603–11.

Stanley, S. (2000) Commentary: the cultural impact of Islam on the future of direction of nurse education. *Nurse Education Today*, **20**(1), 69.

Swinton, J. (2001) *A Space to Listen: Meeting the Spiritual Needs of People with Learning Disabilities*. The Foundation for People with Learning Disabilities, London.

Swinton, J. and Narayanasamy, A. (2002) JAN Forum: Response to: 'A critical view of spirituality and spiritual assessment' by Draper P and McSherry W (2002) [Journal of Advanced Nursing 39: 1–2]. *Journal of Advanced Nursing*, **40**(2), 158–60.

Tanyi, R. A. (2002) Towards clarification of the meaning of spirituality. *Journal of Advanced Nursing*, **39**(5), 500–9.

Utley, A. (2003) Doubting Thomases turn eyes to new age. *The Times Higher Education Supplement*. http://www.asanas.org.uk/.

Waterman, H., Tillen, D., Dickson, R. and de Koning, K. (2001) Action Research: A systematic review and guidance for assessment. *Health Technology Assessment*, **5**(23), 1–166.

CHAPTER 2

Spirituality and health care

Aru Narayanasamy and Mani Narayanasamy

Summary

In this chapter the various aspects of spirituality and health care are reviewed in the context of the literature. In so doing, the concepts of spirituality and religion are examined and this is followed by an exploration of the debates surrounding spirituality in health care. It is acknowledged that a scientific definition of spirituality remains elusive and that post-modern thinkers appear to be accommodating the pluralistic nature of spirituality. There then follows an exploration of spiritual needs and spiritual care.

Key points

- Holistic care is about care of the body, mind and spirit.
- There is a connection between spirituality and healing.
- Spirituality is not necessarily the same as religion.
- Spiritual and religious dimensions of care are important in a pluralistic society.
- Spiritual care interventions benefit patients and staff.

Introduction

Many in the nursing profession have taken pride in their holistic approach to care, that is, caring for the whole person: the body, mind and spirit. Emerging research suggests that spirituality is integral to our wellbeing. Fry (1997) views humans as spiritual beings and adds: 'spirituality is a profound and central aspect of the existence of many people'. In this respect spirituality and nursing are intertwined in the life experience of people. Since nursing involves being a companion to patients' journeys in coping with their ill health and suffering, this point will be developed later in this chapter.

The significance of spirituality and religious beliefs was illustrated in a recent MORI poll. This poll found that three in five Britons (60%) believe in God. One in five British people (18%) claimed to be a practising member of an organised religion, with a quarter (25%) non-practising members (MORI, 2003). A further quarter (24%) are spiritually inclined but do not really have allegiance to any organised religion, while 14% are agnostic and 12% are atheist. This finding has clear implications for health care, as patients may require nurses to respond with sensitivity to their spiritual needs. Jacik (1986) described the nurse's role as an 'inspiriting' one, providing a sense of identity, worth, hope and purpose in existence. It is an 'inspiriting one' for both patients and nurses as both experience a shared communion of relationship in which healing and growth takes place.

Furthermore, there is a consensus of opinion among scholars (Narayana-samy, 2004; Baldacchino, 2003; MacKinlay, 2001; Swinton, 2001; Koenig, 2000; Post and Puchalski, 2000) that spirituality is important for our very existence. Equally, many scholars claim that there is an abundance of evidence to support that spirituality is important to our wellbeing and healing (Larson *et al.*, 1992; Sherwood, 2000). There is also the recognition in medicine of the importance of spirituality, in that there is a revival of interest in the priest-physician role. Research on prayer, as a powerful medicine of healing, is adding to the thinking in medicine (Dossey, 1993). Clearly this evidence is apparent enough for nurses and other health carers to give serious consideration to spirituality (with or without religion) and include it as fundamental part of holistic care. David Aldridge (2000) claims that if nurses ignore spiritual concerns, then they are denying part of patients' very existence.

However, there is evidence to suggest that nurses and health carers are unable to meet the spiritual needs of their patients for a variety of reasons. Many nurses do not fully understand what spirituality means (Ross, 1997; McSherry, 2000). One explanation may be that the word *spirituality* is a swampy one, a semantic confusion. Spirituality is often conflated with religion or treated as constructs depicting the ethereal. Furthermore, it is suggested that the lack of a scientific definition of spirituality has added to this misunderstanding (McSherry and Watson, 2002). There is also a certain degree of ambiguity surrounding the concept of spirituality, in that it is treated as synonymous with religion (Baldacchino, 2003; Sherwood, 2000). Such blurring of the concept has not helped. Others identify a range of barriers acting against spiritual care in health care (Narayanasamy *et al.*, 2002; see Table 2.1).

Table 2.1 Barriers to the provision of spiritual care (adapted from Narayanasamy *et al.* (2002)).

■ Failure to recognise the significance of spirituality in the patients.

■ Carers lack of confidence within this area ,

■ Uncertainty among care providers regarding personal spiritual and religious beliefs and values

■ Embarrassment over the apparently non-scientific nature of spirituality

What is spirituality?

Spirituality may be defined as 'the essence of our being and it gives meaning and purpose to our existence' (Narayanasamy, 2004). The spiritual dimension may further be described as follows (Swinton, 2001; Narayanasamy, 2001; Sherwood, 2000). Our spirituality gives us a sense of personhood and individuality. It is the guiding force behind our uniqueness and acts as an inner source of power and energy, which makes us 'tick over' as a person. Spirituality is the inner, intangible dimension that motivates us to be connected with others and our surrounding. It drives us to search for meaning and purpose, and to establish positive and trusting relationship with others. There is a mysterious nature to our spirituality and it gives peace and tranquillity through our relationship with 'something other' or things we value as supreme. Our spirituality sets us on a journey as part of our growth and development. It provides us with a sense of wholeness, stability, wellness, security, hope and peace. Spirituality can be an important source of wisdom, inspiration, meaning and purpose. It comes into focus at critical junctures in our lives when we face emotional stress, physical illness or death.

Religion

So much has been said about spirituality that it may be useful at this juncture to look at the differences between spirituality and religion. For most of us the word *religion* tends to create images in our minds of external things like buildings, religious officials, and public rituals, such as baptisms, weddings and funerals. For some individuals these are times when they come into contact with something to do with religion, with or without a deeper religious significance. In the literature religions are often described as to do with a supernatural or divine force, a system of beliefs, a comprehensive code of ethics or philosophy or a prescribed set of practices to be followed. Religions are also associated with institutional and symbolic things such as places of worship, religious arte- facts and so on (Swinton, 2001; Murray and Zentner, 1989). However, there is consensus that spirituality is much broader than religion. Spirituality usually signifies much more abstract aspects of humanity, including areas such as the meaning of life, love, humanity, inner peace, tranquillity, meditation, relation- ships, individuality, personal worth and so on.

Spirituality is usually treated as a subjective dimension, implicit in nature, inward-focused and having to do with feelings and experiences, a personal entity, and a form of journey. In contrast, religion is viewed as a concrete dimension that is explicit and outward-looking, related to objective things like institutions, religious buildings and so on. For some people religion is a mode of transport for their spiritual journey.

Some people may be highly spiritual in nature but not necessarily religious, while others may be religious without being spiritual. However, some people may use religion as a medium to express their spirituality and as a way of relat- ing to the transcendent (MacKinlay, 2001). Spirituality is more of a journey, and religion may become the transport to help us in our journey.

Although there is evidence that membership of established mainstream churches has dropped dramatically, it is now estimated that there may be as many as 12,000 new religious groups in the UK (Brierley, 2000). Opinions vary about the popular- ity of the new religious groups. One view is that this may be due to the spiritual void that many people may be experiencing because of the declining popularity of established religious institutions. Others suggest it is a feature of postmodern- ism and consumerism, where people are simply exercising their right to pick and mix products, including spirituality and religion, as commodities. Aldridge (2003), in his writing on consumerism, implies that spirituality has become a commod- ity or cultural product in consumption-orientated postmodern society. The spiritual need for searching for meaning and purpose may act as an intangible motivator for membership of New Religious Movements (NRMs). Wallis (1984) categorises the emerging new religions and the revival of the traditional ones into new religious movements. According to Wallis (1984) the NRMs fall into two categories:

- World-affirming movements
- World-rejecting movements

World-affirming movements

World-affirming movements are usually individualistic and life-positive, and aim to release human potentials. They may not have a church or central place of worship as such, or a developed theology or ethics. They accept the world as it is, but enable individual members to participate more effectively and gain more from their worldly experience. The world-affirming movements claim to offer opportunities for members to access spiritual or supernatural powers, and in this regard they could be regarded as religious. Members are not normally required to change their lifestyle and behaviour, but they offer the followers the potential to be successful in terms of their society's values and norms by unlocking the spiritual powers within the individual. Followers are believed to be capable of achieving salvation through personal achievement. Members are usually supported to overcome personal problems, such as unhappiness, suffering or disability, by adopting techniques that heighten their awareness or abilities. World-affirming movements do not normally attempt to convert or proselytise for new members; instead they sell their services commercially. Membership includes mainly the middle class. For example, Scientology as a world-affirming movement, has a number of high-profile members including John Travolta and Tom Cruise. Members are not subject to strict social controls and defaulters are not usually excluded. Transcendental Meditation (TM) is considered to be another world-affirming movement. It gained popularity when the Beatles were introduced to its leading proponent, the Maharishi Mahesh Yogi, in 1968. According to Bruce (1995), TM, as an Eastern product, has been tailored for Western sensibilities.

World-rejecting movements

World-rejecting movements are highly critical of the outside world and demand significant commitment from their members, especially to make active changes to their lives. They expect members to pray and study religious texts and follow strong ethical codes. They are exclusive and often share possessions, and group identity is important. They are often Millenarian, which means expecting divine intervention to change the world. The world-rejecting movements vary in size; some, such as the Unification Church, have international membership, whilst others have smaller memberships. Some world-rejecting movements act as total institutions and exert greater control over the lives of their members. Consequently, allegations have been made against these movements' reputation for 'brainwashing' adherents, since people who had been close to individuals, including families and friends, find that they have changed psychologically beyond recognition. Such concerns have led to controversies and scandals in the media about the cult status of some world-rejecting movements.

The negative publicity surrounding cults may have an impact upon caring professionals with regard to meeting the spiritual needs of their members. Some staff may feel ambivalent towards a patient belonging to certain movements with cult status. In such situations, it is paramount to explore the best ethical way of responding to such members' spiritual needs. No matter how difficult it is, spiritual care is about 'loving the stranger' in the midst of their health crisis, and it is always the best interest of the patients that should be served. Whatever label an individual carries, there is always an individual with a spirit behind it. If the health professional feels ill-equipped to deal with patients' spiritual needs, then the advice of the Department of Spiritual and Pastoral Care or the patient's religious representative should be sought. Even if there is a delay in seeking advice, health care professionals still have a duty to care. They need to respond in a caring, compassionate and non-judgmental manner in addressing the holistic needs of their patients.

Although some NRMs reject or accept materialism, they all have a focus on spiritual and personal empowerment. The increasing popularity of spirituality means that it has become commodified and marketed as a product in consumer societies. There are now large sections in bookshops devoted to the literature on NRMs, which signify their popularity. There is huge market potential for products to enhance our wellbeing in terms of our body, mind and spirit. High street shops and supermarkets offer packaged products in response to consumers' need to look after their body, mind and spirit.

Current debates on spirituality and health care

The 2003 MORI poll casts doubts on the claim that Britain is a secular society. Indeed, such claims may now be regarded as a myth. There is emerging literature that attempts to address the subject of spiritual nursing and a multifaith society (MacLaren, 2004). Furthermore, there is a consensus of opinions among scholars (Narayanasamy, 2004; MacKinlay, 2001; Swinton, 2001; Koenig, 2000; Post and Puchalski, 2000) that spirituality is the essence of our being and gives meaning and purpose to our very existence. Equally, many scholars provide ample evidence to support that spirituality is important to our wellbeing and healing (Larson *et al.*, 1992; Sherwood, 2000). Another breakthrough is the renaissance in medicine about the importance of spirituality, in that there is a revival of interest in the priest-physician role. Such evidence is compelling enough to argue that nurses and other health carers should give serious consideration to spirituality (with or without religion) and include it as a fundamental part of nursing. That is, they should provide truly holistic care (care of the body, mind and spirit).

Emerging directions in spirituality

Several authors provide useful directions on spirituality in the broad sense (MacLaren, 2004; Baldacchino, 2003; Aldridge, 2000). These authors suggest that spiritual care as a paradigm is necessary for health care in the context of multifaith Britain. In response to the important editorial commentary on spirituality in the *Journal of Advanced Nursing* by Draper and McSherry (2002), Swinton and Narayanasamy (2002) highlight the universality and enduring nature of spirituality pervading humanity. However, some authors give the impression that there is a lack of clarity of what is meant by spirituality. If it is seen from a narrow worldview of nursing, then there is a blurring of the concept. This is partly because of Northern American religious (mainly Christian evangelical) perspectives of spirituality, and partly because of the lack of epistemological awareness in nursing in terms of philosophy (mainly existentialism) and theology. Discourses originating from philosophy and theology provide many insights into the evolving constructions of the concept of spirituality and shifting epistemological instances of this subject matter. Drawing from theology, Bradshaw (1994) advances that the classical theological position 'has shown to define the spirituality dimension of man as the essence of his person, not differentiated from his physicality or psychology, and inextricably linked to his relationship with God' (p. 16). Baldacchino (2003) utilises the cognitive stress-coping theory (Lazarus and Folkman, 1984) and the numinous experience (Otto, 1950) to develop her discourse on spirituality in illness and care.

More recently, Henery (2003) pointed out that there is a lack of in-depth analysis of the concept of spirituality in nursing. However, although her work is largely based on Christian theology of spirituality and spiritual care, Bradshaw (1994) provides a comprehensive treatment of this subject by drawing from theology and philosophy, including existentialism. Equally, if one is looking for a clear discourse on spirituality in nursing, they can find it in the work of MacKinlay (2001). Elizabeth MacKinlay attempts to map the spiritual dimension of a number of independent living elders. Through stories from participants she illuminates how spiritual health in ageing can be enhanced by sensitising older people to their own spiritual journey. Baldacchino (2003) provides a comprehensive view of spirituality in the light of her research work with patients in Malta. Although the study's sample comprised largely Catholics, Baldacchino's findings illuminate the importance of spiritual coping mechanisms, such as the relationship with God and prayers among Maltese patients as they faced challenges of acute illnesses, such as myocardial infarctions. Clearly, Baldacchino adds to the discourse on transcultural spirituality. There need to be further discourses of such nature in nursing and health care.

The search for a scientific notion of spirituality

It seems that one major obstacle to a common definition of spirituality is the search for a scientific notion of spirituality. The preoccupation with establishing scientific credibility in nursing means that there is intense pressure to subject spirituality to rigorous investigative procedures to construct a scientific notion of spirituality that is free from ambiguity. However, this remains elusive as there is evidence to suggest that spirituality as a concept is not easily amenable to definitions or measurements (Aldridge, 2000; Swinton, 2001). Aldridge (2000, p. 36) asserts that 'It [spirituality] is ineffable and totally subjective, making itself elusive to scientific inquiry'. Likewise, Swinton (2001, p. 13) argues that spirituality is 'not easy to analyse and conceptualise in the language of science'. Consequently, spirituality is marginalised. However, science has not provided answers to many causes of diseases and their cure. For this and other reasons, in the postmodern world science is losing credibility and is viewed as contestable in many of its claims.

Postmodernism is challenging the meta-narratives of science, philosophy, theology and other related disciplines (Burr, 2003). Although contested by some, there is a claim that we now live in a postmodern world. Postmodernism marks the decline of trust in the credibility of science and faith in technological progress. Woods (1999, p. 11) describes postmodernism as representing the:

> decline of faith in the keystones of the Enlightenment – belief in the infinite progress of knowledge, belief in infinite moral and social advancement, belief in teleology – and its rigorous definition of the standards of intelligibility, coherence and legitimacy

The challenge to meta-narratives and other discourses is due to disillusionment with the monopoly of science, religion or grand political schemes like Marxism (Butler, 2002). This disillusionment has pushed us into an era where personal stories and competing theories are equally valued. Provisional rather than universal and absolute forms of legitimisation are welcome. There is also a belief that knowledge can only be partial, fragmented and incomplete. The emphasis in postmodernism is placed upon the social construction of identities, in opposition to essentialism, which seeks to locate identities in physical and cultural realities. Identity is seen as fluid and multiple, reflecting the various life courses of social exposure that individuals undertake.

However, we are not taking a position that is antagonistic to positivism. On the contrary, spirituality can be subjected to scientific study, but we may have to reframe our way of thinking about science to 'accommodate for the new perspectives that science brings to us' (Swinton, 2001, p. 13). Science and technology are playing a crucial role in establishing the scientific basis of spirituality. Newberg *et al.*'s (2002) scientific study using sophisticated scanning techniques is providing neurological evidence supporting the universal presence of spirituality in human beings, which they claim is there for an evolutionary purpose (Swinton and Narayanasamy, 2002). Other studies designed to evoke spiritual experiences in laboratory conditions are being attempted with inconclusive results. However, a definite scientific theory of spirituality has yet to emerge. This may be because of the mysterious nature of spirituality and spiritual experiences. Sir Alistair Hardy (1987) and Hay (1987) recount the numinous (Otto, 1950) and mysterious (James, 1983) nature of spirituality in their empirical studies of spiritual experiences in the general population. Rudolf Otto described the numinous in terms of a positive (fascinans) or negative (awe-fulness) experience that happens to individuals, which is considered to be Divine in origin. Baldacchino (2003, p. xxiii) further explains the numinous experience derived from Otto (1950) in the context of illness and suffering:

> The numinous experience refers to a complex feeling state of personal insufficient, longing to reach a higher power to find existential meaning. The numen exists as an inborn capacity which can be induced or awakened to enable the individual to find existential meaning. Thus, during the crisis situation, an individual transcends beyond the self to relate to god, resulting in empowerment and ability to cope with illness.

James (1983) describes the mysterious nature of spiritual experiences felt by some individuals as noetic, transient, ineffable and passivity. It is most likely that the numinous and mysterious nature of spirituality makes it elusive to definitions, as each one of these experiences is unique and ineffable. James describes in detail the mysterious nature of spirituality in his book *The Varieties of Religious Experience*. He recounts that spiritual experiences manifest in a variety of forms. He attributed four qualities to spiritual experiences:

1. Noetic: described as something new and unique, and qualitatively beyond the bounds of normal human experience.
2. Ineffability: individuals described the ineffable nature of their experience which was difficult to translate it into human terms.
3. Transient: the experience was transient in that it lasted for a short duration. It was sudden and lasted for seconds.
4. Passivity: individuals described that when they went through the experience they felt as if being taken over by something beyond their control.

Returning to the theme of spirituality and health care, to dismiss or ignore its significance in the caring context on the basis that it lacks clarity and scientific credibility is a gross injustice to humanity and could be damaging to the essence of our being. The philosopher G. E. Moore, in his seminal work on intuitionism, once said that the terms 'yellow' or 'good' are indefinable, yet we do not deny their existence but allow them to pervade our lives (Bowie, 2001). But why do we question that part of us (inner dimension/essence of our being), when many unequivocally accept its existence. Many of us rely on our cars to make journeys, but we may not necessarily understand how the engine works. We do not stop driving our cars because we do not know how the engine works or what is under its bonnet. Likewise, spirituality is important for our journey in helping us to search for meaning, purpose, hope, connectedness, harmony, peace, love, beauty, ecstasy, trust, reality and so on. We do not necessarily need to understand what it is and its intricacies to help others when spirituality 'comes into focus when an individual faces emotional distress, illness or death' (Murray and Zentner, 1989). In my view, spirituality is spirituality – we know intuitively that it is within us, and *that is the end of the matter*, as G. E. Moore would put it.

Can there be a consensus on the notion of spirituality?

There is an impression that nurses neglect to recognise patients' spirituality because there is a lack of consensus with regard to the definition of spirituality. However, contemporary scholars, such as Aldridge (2000), Sherwood (2000), MacKinlay (2001) and Swinton (2001), to name a few, clarify the concept of spirituality. Most notably, Aldridge charts 17 definitions of spirituality which converge on the point about the multidimensional nature of spirituality and that it is to do with unity and meaning, and transcendence. Readers are advised to consult Aldridge (2000) for details about the definitions of spirituality in terms of meaning and transcendence.

Jessica MacLaren (2004) alludes to the point that relatively little nursing research has been done on this topic and paints a gloomy picture with regard to the poor quality of some of the research on spiritual coping strategies (Baldacchino and Draper, 2001). However, it is not clear what criteria have been used to draw such conclusions. Emerging qualitative research findings highlight the significance of spiritual care and its healing effects upon patients and carers. Swinton (2001) provides qualitative evidence on the lived experience of mental health clients and their spirituality, while MacKinlay (2001) provides illuminating accounts of the spiritual experiences in older people. Likewise, Ross (1997) highlights the significance of spiritual care of older patients and Narayanasamy (2002) describes the findings of a qualitative study on spiritual coping mechanisms in chronically ill patients. Across the Atlantic, Sherwood (2000) identifies patients' spiritual needs through empirical research. Matthews (1998), Koenig (2000) and Dossey (1993) provide both qualitative and quantitative data derived from well-designed empirical studies to amplify the centrality of spirituality and spiritual practices, both secular and non-secular, in healing and promotion of wellbeing.

Furthermore, in the UK Ross (1997), McSherry (2000) and Narayanasamy and Owen (2001) provide evidence of nurses' involvement in spiritual care in the broad sense. Mary O'Brien (2003) draws from various empirical studies of spirituality in clinical practice to develop the themes for her book on spiritual care. Also, Ross (1997), Narayanasamy and Owen (2001) and Narayanasamy *et al*. (2002) have began to map out what nurses do when they claim to provide spiritual care. The findings from the studies by Narayanasamy and Owen (2001) and Narayanasamy *et al*. (2002) are reported in Chapters 5 and 6, respectively.

Spirituality is a private and inner dimension

However, there is a trend emerging in nursing that is dismissive of the importance of spirituality in the clinical context on the basis of a small number of findings that suggest patients are unable to articulate what spirituality is in terms of languages familiar to spirituality researchers. Spirituality is a very private, inner matter to most people (Narayanasamy, 2002), and if it is externalised it is done so in terms of metaphors and linguistic patterns that are more in tune with one's culture, symbols, practices and so on (Linbeck, 1984). To be dismissive of the significance of spirituality in health care on the grounds that patients do not use similar languages to those of spirituality researchers equates to professional patronisation and imperialism. We need to avoid adopting the closed system in science, where any attempt to step outside the accepted conventions is usually ignored or rejected; this happened, for example, in the move from Newtonian to Einsteinian physics. Deepak Chopra (1989), the much acclaimed writer on spirituality who brings a blend of Eastern and Western thinking to almost all of his works on spirituality and healing observes: 'science has accepted essentially a frozen, geometric way of mapping out everything that happens in the material world...' (p. 50). Preconceptions and assumptions about patients' spirituality and spiritual needs must be suspended until a fuller picture is available through extensive studies of this phenomenon. The way forward is through a more open system of inquiry to capture the lived experience of the phenomenon of spirituality in health and illness. As postmodernists would put it, there is a need for more narratives of spirituality from patients. There is a need to deconstruct the grand narratives of science by transgression – we need to cross over boundaries to understand fully patients' narratives of their spirituality. This means being open-minded, freeing ourselves from the narrow confines of science, removing our professional veil and entering patients' worlds by getting them to tell their stories – their versions of events – capturing realities. However, some nursing authors show overoptimism when the term 'postmodern nursing' is used. In my view, nursing is caught between modernism and postmodernism. In its efforts to be seen as scientifically credible, there appears to be a reluctance to be engaged in the arduous task of deconstructing the meta-narratives of science, including spirituality and religions. If it happens, the scholarship in nursing remains modest and sporadic with respect to the discourse on spirituality.

The call for pluralism in approaches to spirituality

Some authors (Narayanasamy, 2004; Kissane, 2004) argue that there needs to be a pluralistic approach to spiritual care, as Britain is a multicultural and multifaith society. Maclaren (2004) provides a perspective on multifaith and secularism, but appears to marginalise Hinduism by locating it among developing spheres of spirituality, for example New Age spirituality and so on. Some may regard this as a form of cultural imperialism in which eastern spirituality is trivialised. Deepak Chopra (2000) and other sources (Parrinder, 1968; Fellow, 1978; Scott Littleton, 1996; Smart, 1996) observe that Hinduism predates other institutional religions and they illustrate that it (whether seen as a religion or way of life) has well-developed spirituality. Hinduism is a western concept (etic) to describe a way of life, but an emic point of view; Indians talk about the Vedic religion instead of Hinduism. In the main, Hinduism is pluralistic and normally tolerant of other religions and has no founder; nor does it involve initiation rites (baptism) to be a Hindu. In relative terms all religious practices and New Age spiritualities converge with regard to mysticism and meditation, a strong feature of Hinduism (or Vedanta). There is a need to address Islam, Hinduism and Sikhism to enhance the discourse on spirituality in health care in the United Kingdom. Religion plays a significant role among British minority ethnic communities of Muslims, Sikhs and Hindus (Narayanasamy, 2004).

The concern in the literature about the lack of guidance on how to meet the needs of multifaiths is addressed, to some extent, in the excellent resource material by Henley and Schott (1999) and Holland and Hogg (2001). The ASSET and ACCESS Models (see Narayanasamy and Andrews, 2000) offer a framework for meeting the spiritual and cultural needs of patients. One of the major barriers to the provision of adequate spiritual care in practice is to do with values. With regard to values, if nurses and health carers are not fully self-aware of their own spirituality, then they are unlikely to be sensitive to the spiritual needs of others. The importance of value clarifications related to personal beliefs and values through a self-awareness programme is well documented in the literature (Parfitt, 1998; McSherry, 2000; Swinton, 2001).

Spiritual needs

There are variations in the way spiritual needs are described in the literature (Baldacchino, 2003; MacKinlay, 2001; Narayanasamy, 2001; McSherry, 2000; Shelly, 2000). Spiritual needs may be attained through meaning and purpose, loving and harmonious relationships, forgiveness, hope and strength, trust and personal beliefs and values, spiritual practices, concept of God/Deity, beliefs and practices, and creativity. These are explored further.

The need for meaning and purpose, love and relatedness and forgiveness

Several authors identify the need for meaning and purpose, the need for love and relatedness and the need for forgiveness as features of spiritual needs (O'Brien, 2003; Narayanasamy, 2001; McSherry, 2000; Shelly, 2000; Shelly and Fish, 1988; Highfields and Cason, 1983). According to McSherry, Shelly and Fish appear to be taking a Judeo-Christian approach to spirituality. However, the literature suggests that the search for meaning is a primary force in life. This drives us to search for meaning to life in general and discovering meaning in suffering in particular. We need to make sense of our life and illness. Patients requiring medical interventions may find new meaning and purpose during the trajectory of their illness. There is evidence to suggest that patients struggle with finding a source of meaning and purpose in their lives (Narayanasamy, 2002). It is suggested that people with a sense of meaning and purpose survive more readily in very difficult circumstances, and these include illness and suffering. There is some truth in the expression that he who has a 'why' to life can bear with almost any 'how' (Frankl, 1987).

Many of us approach the task of life in a variety of ways, so our ability to cope with a crisis varies. We can find meaning and purpose in the experience of suffering. There is a distinction between the religious and the apparently non-religious person in the way they approach spirituality: that is, religious persons experience their existence not merely as a task, but as a mission, and are aware of their taskmaster, the source of their mission. That source is God (O'Brien, 2003). Writing from a theological perspective, Warren (2002) argues that our meaning maker is God, and Christians will find meaning and purpose through their relationship with Jesus Christ. Warren claims 'Without God, life has no meaning, and without purpose, life has no meaning. Without meaning, life has no significance or hope' (p. 30).

Critical junctures in life, such as illness, trauma and loss, may throw a person into a state of meaninglessness; that is, the person expresses a sense of bewilderment and loss of meaning (Narayanasamy, 2002; Aldridge, 2000). Fear, anger, anxiety and a sense of poor self-concept are some of the psychological factors that may affect the person in crisis. For example, the person at the end of life may cry out for help in search of meaning and desperately seek to talk to someone who will give attention and time to their exploration of meaning and purpose. Uncertainty evokes fear, discomfort, pain and suffering (Coyle, 2002). The nurse is very often the nearest person to whom sufferers can reach out.

In a person searching for meaning and purpose there may be a need for exploration of spiritual and psychological issues. In some instances the person in search of spirituality may want to talk about religious feelings or a lack of them. The person may not be asking advice or opinions but just for an opportunity to talk about feelings, to express doubts and anguish. Such opportunity for expression can bring about clarity and a renewed sense of meaning, purpose and hope. According to Coyle (2002), spirituality 'motivates, enables, empowers, and provides hope'.

People who have strong religious convictions and sense God still need encouragement to adapt to unexpected changes. They are likely to experience hope even when their usual support systems let them down. Their experience of God reassures them that God will never fail them. The nurse may have to act as a catalyst in providing the opportunity for finding meaning and purpose. During the crisis of illness the nurse may help patients to establish their relationship with God.

The human need for love and relatedness (harmonious relationships) goes hand in hand with a need for meaning and purpose (Narayanasamy, 2001). The needs for love and to give love are fundamental human needs (Maslow, 1968) throughout our lives. Deepak Chopra (1997) epitomises love as central to our lives and highlights its healing properties. Using a blend of eastern mysticism and western medicine, Chopra makes remarkable claims about love as a spiritual resource in mending our brokenness to regain our wholeness as a person. He aptly declares, 'Love is spirit. Spirit is love' (p. 33). Indeed, Chopra has devoted a whole book, *The Path to Love* to the spiritual significance of love.

There is evidence to suggest that the spiritually distressed person also experiences an intense sense of estrangement, and possibly feels alienated and disconnected from outside relationships as well as within the clinical environment (Narayanasamy, 2002). The need for unconditional love becomes paramount as a way of reconnecting with others. Although unconditional love may be a universal experience, a spiritually distressed person requires more of this – that is, love that has no strings attached to it. This is sometimes referred to as 'in spite of' love (Narayanasamy, 2001; Bradshaw, 1994). The spiritually and psychological distressed person does not have to earn it by being good or attractive or wealthy. The person is simply loved for the way he or she is, regardless of faults or ignorance or bad habits or deeds.

The manifestations of the need for love are self-pity, depression, insecurity, isolation and fear. These are indicators of a need for love from oneself, other people and, if the person is religious, God. The person receiving this kind of love experiences feelings of self-worth, joy, security, belonging, hope and courage. The spiritually distressed person also has a need to give love and be free from worries, which may include, for example, worries about the financial status of the family during hospitalisation/separation from family and worries about separation from others during death.

Forgiveness can be seen from two sides: the need to give and receive. A person who experiences spiritual distress expresses feelings of guilt and therefore requires the opportunity for forgiveness. Some people seek forgiveness through prayers. Guilt often emerges when a person experiences the realisation that one has failed to live up to his or her own expectations or the expectations of others.

Guilt may manifest as feelings of paranoia, hostility, worthlessness, defensiveness, withdrawal, psychosomatic complaints, rationalisations, criticism of self, others and God, and 'scapegoating'. Evidence shows that forgiveness may bring a feeling of joy, peace and elation, and a sense of renewed self worth (Macaskill, 2002; Narayanasamy, 2001). Confession of sin is one way in which some people achieve forgiveness from God. A recent study on forgiveness by Macaskill (2002) suggests that those who forgive also derive positive effects in terms of healing.

Hope and strength, trust and creativity

Highfields and Cason (1983) and Narayanasamy (2001) identify the following as spiritual needs: hope and strength, trust and creativity. For many of us our sense of hope can be a powerful motivator in enabling an open attitude toward new ways of coping. The spiritually distressed person may experience a feeling of hopelessness. The hopeless person may see no way out; there may be no other possibilities other than those dreaded.

We thrive on good relationships with others, and this is another facet of our hope (Narayanasamy, 2001). These includes relationships with others, ourselves and the world, what a person believes and what is desired is possible. Hope is also necessary for future plans. Further sources of our hope include seeking support, love and the stability provided by important relationships in our life, and putting into action future plans. If the patient believes in God, then hope in God is important. For believers, this hoping in God is the ultimate source of strength and supersedes all aspirations that are transitional.

Hope is closely related to our need for a source of strength. A source of hope provides the spiritual and psychological strength that we may need. A source of strength gives us the courage needed to face innumerable odds in a crisis. Haase's (1987) study found that the subjects concurred that belief in the power of prayer helped them cope with medical procedures, and opportunities to express their faith helped them to resolve the situation they described. For some, communication with God and prayer is a source of strength. More recent studies suggest similar findings (Narayanasamy, 2002; Koenig, 2001; Thomsen, 1998; Benson and Stark, 1996).

Many of us feel secure when we can establish a trusting relationship with others. The spiritually distressed patient requiring medical interventions needs an environment that conveys a trusting relationship. Such an environment is one which demonstrates that carers make themselves accessible to others, both physically and emotionally. Trusting is the ability to place confidence in the trustworthiness of others and this is essential for spiritual health and total well-being. Learning to trust in an environment which is alien can be a daunting task and is not an easy skill to accomplish. A trusting friendship and support may help patients to put themselves on track for spiritual wellness.

Spiritual practices, concept of God or Deity, and creativity

The opportunity to express needs related to spiritual practices, the concept of God or Deity, and creativity may present as a feature of spirituality during illness. For some the concept of God or Deity may be an important function in the inner life. The need to carry out spiritual practices concerning God or Deity may be too daunting for the person if the opportunity is not available or the environment is alien or unreceptive to this need. For some, creative needs may feature. Meditation, relaxation, creation of personal space and creative pursuits may help the spiritually distressed to come out of their current predicament.

Personal beliefs and values

The opportunity to express personal beliefs and values is a known spiritual need (Narayanasamy, 2001). In this sense, spirituality refers to anything that a person considers to be of highest value in life. Religious practices may provide opportunities for shared expression of personal beliefs through corporate worship and prayers. For some, contact with fellow believers can be an important source of support. Personal values which may be highly regarded by an individual include, for example, beliefs of a formalised religious path, whereas for others such values might be a set of very personal philosophical statements, or perhaps a physical activity.

Spiritual care

Numerous authors offer strategies for spiritual care (Ross, 1998; Govier, 2000; McSherry, 2000; Narayanasamy, 2001; Swinton, 2001). Writing from a mental health perspective, using a phenomenological approach, Swinton suggests that a multidisciplinary approach to spiritual care is desirable. In particular, he argues that assessment of the person's spirituality and the implementation of an appropriate form of spiritual care requires not only in-depth interviews, but also a collaboration of disciplines. Nurses, chaplains, social workers, occupational therapists, family and friends can all provide invaluable information. The client is the central person here. However, Swinton observes that nurses are ideally placed to assess and understand the role of spirituality in those in their care. In this regard, nurses can provide a therapeutic presence that can empower and enable change. Goldberg (1998) refers to this kind of intervention as 'presencing' and points out its benefits to patients. In developing a discourse on presencing derived from Roach (1991), Goldberg writes 'providing a presence which empowers and enables others to change, to accept, to grow, to die peacefully, is what nurses do each day' (p. 838). Moreover, in a phenomenological study of nurses' experiences, Dunniece and Slevin (2000, p. 614) suggest that 'presence' or 'being there' includes 'giving information, explaining, answering questions, listening and simply being present without speaking'. These authors provide evidence from their own study and others that the phenomenon of 'presence' or 'being there' is important in the care of cancer patients. However, they note that 'being there' is more than a physical presence.

Nursing practice

Several authors offer other strategies for spiritual care (Ross, 1997; McSherry, 2000; Narayanasamy, 2001; O'Brien, 2003). These are discussed next. A problem-based approach should be used systematically to plan care to meet the spiritual needs of their patients (Narayanasamy, 2001). Mary O'Brien (2003) observes that some nurses may feel unprepared or reluctant to discuss spiritual or religious topics with patients and suggests that a systematic approach to assessing spiritual wellbeing is recommended. Nursing concentration on helping patients in their growth can lead to improvements in patients' overall wellbeing. There is an emphasis in the literature that the primary purpose of spiritual care is to help the person suffering from sickness or disability to attain or maintain peace of mind. The following strategies may be used for spiritual care (McSherry, 2000).

Assessing spiritual needs

Valuable information central to spiritual needs should be obtained from patients. However, McSherry and Ross (2002) argue that assessing spiritual needs can be problematic, since there is a lack of consensus about what spirituality means. They observe that the word 'spirituality' lacks a common set of defining characteristics as it means different things to different people. Following a review of the subject in the literature, McSherry and Ross conclude that in spite of the popular debates about what it is and what it is not, the concept is clouded by more misconception, ambiguity and subjectivity than ever before. Many of the existing assessment tools are designed to measure practice factors, which are amenable to precise definitions and measurement. However, spirituality remains elusive to precise definition and measurement because many of its attributes are mysterious, personal and private in nature, as suggested earlier. Furthermore, other tools (for example, Stoll's (1979) guidelines for spiritual assessment) are suited for religious needs assessment rather than spiritual needs.

Narayanasamy (2001) offers an assessment guide which may help with the gathering of information to establish spiritual needs (see Table 2.2). This tool appears to be compatible with Catterall *et al.*'s (1998, p. 4) suggestion that assessment guidelines should be 'easy to use, flexible and take little time to assess the spiritual state of patients at different times and in different situations'.

McSherry and Ross (2002) call for a greater degree of sensitivity and flexibility, and the use of appropriate language when using spiritual assessment instruments as a way of resolving potential problems such as Judeo-Christian bias, intrusiveness and accusation of unsolicited interventions involving spirituality, which for many people is a very private, personal and inner thing. Other spiritual assessment tools are found in O'Brien (2003), McSherry and Ross (2002), Govier (2000); Swinton (2001), Farran *et al.* (1998) and Maugan (1996).

Formulating care plans

The information from the application of above assessment guide may contribute to the formulation of spiritual care plans (Narayanasamy, 2001). When formulating the care plan, careful consideration should be given to the patient's individuality, the willingness of the nurse to get involved in the spirituality of the patient, the use of the therapeutic self, and the nurturing of the inner person (the spirit).

Table 2.2 Spiritual assessment guide.

Needs	Questions	Assessment notes
Meaning and purpose	What gives you a sense of meaning and purpose? Is there anything especially meaningful to you now? Does the patient/client make any sense of illness/suffering? Does the patient/client show any sense of meaning and purpose?	
Sources of strength and hope	Who is the most important person to you? To whom would you turn to when you need help? Is there anyone we can contact? In what ways do they help? What is your source of strength and hope? What helps you the most when you feel afraid or need special help?	
Love and relatedness	How does patient relate to: Family and relatives Friends Others Surrounding Does patient/client appear peaceful? What gives patient/client peace?	
Self-esteem	Describe the state of client/patient's self-esteem How does patient/client feel about self?	
Fear and anxiety	Is patient/client fearful/anxious about anything? Is there anything that alleviates fear/anxiety?	
Anger	Is patient/client angry about anything? How does patient/client cope with anger? How does patient/client control this?	
Relation between spiritual beliefs and health	What has bothered you most being sick (or in what is happening to you?) What do you think is going to happen to you?	

Giving spiritual care

Care plans can guide spiritual care intervention based on an action plan which reflects caring for the individual. It is necessary to develop a caring relationship which signifies to the person that he or she is significant. It requires an approach which combines support and assistance in growing spiritually. In order to give spiritual care the following skills are necessary: self-awareness, communication, trust building and giving hope (Narayanasamy, 2001; McSherry, 2000). These are outlined below.

Self-awareness

Self-awareness can be elaborated as an acknowledgement of our:

- values, attitudes, prejudices beliefs, assumptions and feelings
- personal motives and needs and the extent to which these are being met
- degree of attention to others
- genuineness and investment of self, and how those above might have an effect on others, i.e. the intentional and unconscious use of self.

Communication skills

Swinton (2001) suggests that nurses and health carers need to develop the language of spirituality, such as meaning, hope, value, connectedness and transcendence. Mastery of such language leads to therapeutic understanding and the possibility of genuine spiritual care becomes a reality.

The rudiments of communication skills include:

- active listening without being judgmental
- showing genuineness and unconditional acceptance of clients
- creating the right climate for clients to express spiritual thoughts and feelings

Trust building

- showing genuine concern and giving attention to clients enhances trust and promotes a sense of security
- being reliable and keeping promises made to clients to adhere to care plans and carry them out promptly

Giving hope

- showing humility and humour
- enabling clients to maximise their potential, worth and talents

- working with clients to reaffirm their faith, if required; this gives them hope and strength
- enabling clients to uplift their good memories

Being a catalyst for the client's spiritual growth

- share and learn about each other's spirituality
- giving attention to clients according to the points identified earlier – these will enable spiritual growth for both

Evaluating spiritual care

The final stage of the nursing process is evaluation. Evaluation is an activity that involves the process of making a judgement about the outcomes of medical and health care interventions (Swinton, 2001; Ross, 1998). According to Rousseau (2000), spiritual suffering is 'complex and nebulous and often difficult to assess'. Spiritual suffering may increasingly manifest as physical or psychological problems (Stolley and Koenig, 1997; Kuhn, 1988). According to Swinton, the evaluation process ascertains the efficacy or otherwise of the process, i.e. whether or not spiritual wellbeing is enhanced, distress is increased or decreased, or the situation is unchanged.

According to Narayanasamy (2001), the following questions may be helpful as part of the evaluation process:

- Is the patient's belief system stronger?
- Do the patient's professed beliefs support and direct actions and words?
- Does the patient gain peace and strength from spiritual resources (such as prayer and minister's visits) to face the rigours of treatment, rehabilitation, or peaceful death?
- Does the patient seem more in control and have a clearer self-concept?
- Is the patient at ease in being alone? In having life plans changed?
- Is the patient's behaviour appropriate to the occasion?
- Has reconciliation of any differences taken place between the patient and others?
- Are mutual respect and love obvious in the patient's relationships with others?
- Are there any signs of physical improvement?
- Is there an improved rapport with other patients?

Spiritual integrity is a key indicator of psychological and spiritual support. The person who has attained spiritual integrity and demonstrates this experience through a reality-based tranquillity or peace, or through the development of meaningful, purposeful behaviour, displays a restored sense of integrity. O'Brien (1982) comments that the measure of spiritual care should establish the degree to which 'spiritual pain' was relieved. Another view, offered by Kim *et al.* (1984), suggests that spiritual care may be measured as the disruption in the 'life principle' being restored. The contents of patient's thoughts and feelings may also reflect spiritual growth through a greater understanding of life or through acceptance and creativity within a particular context.

Swinton (2000) develops a discourse to illustrate the usefulness of models of spiritual care, but at the same time raises some serious questions about the nature of such models. In other words, is spiritual care a practical wisdom or 'simply another competency, or is it and foremost a basic principle that underlies our whole approach to mental health care?' (p. 186). Swinton concludes that it may serve both, and in this case it may serve to deal effectively with the competency dimension of spiritual care, although it may remain insufficient in addressing the deeper ontological dimensions of spiritual care. Another criticism is that models of spiritual care may appear to be a mechanistic framework for caring actions rather than a way of being for both with nurse and patient. Sometimes, models and other structured approach to interventions may remove the symmetrical relationship that is desirable in nurse–patient encounters. The connectedness that is necessary in spiritual care is through such relationships, where spiritual growth and transcendence occur naturally and spontaneously rather than in a planned and orderly manner. Also, if spirituality is a state of being and one in which relationships are central to its stability, then should we impose an artificial process such as a model of care, which may actually impede or interfere with a natural human process such as spirituality? Spiritual care may feature as a response to spiritual needs, but it may be *ad hoc*, unplanned, momentary, relational and unpredictable.

However, in spite of the limitations, care models in general offer conceptual frameworks within which health care professionals can systematically gather information on the spiritual lives of patients and provide the support in which spirituality can be a resource that provides healing. Spiritual support is a highly skilful activity. It requires education and experience in spiritual support and care. Sufficient information is provided in the light of research to guide readers on spiritual support and care. It is imperative that the caring team observe the following during health care interventions:

- Do not impose personal beliefs (or lack of them) on patient or families.
- Respond to patient's expression of need with a correct understanding of their background.
- Be sensitive to patient's signal for spiritual support.

If a member of the caring team feels unable to respond to a particular situation of spiritual need, then he or she should then enlist the services of an appropriate individual.

Health care interventions should be based on an action which reflects caring for the individual. There is no cure without caring. Caring signifies to the person that he or she is significant, and is worth someone taking the trouble to be concerned about them. Caring requires actions of support and assistance in growing. It means a non-judgmental approach and showing sensitivity to a person's cultural values, physical preferences and social needs. It demands an attitude of helping, sharing, nurturing and loving.

Conclusion

In this chapter the relationship between spirituality and health was examined in the context of research-based evidence. In doing so, it was established that spirituality is central to healing, and this can be promoted in various ways. A multidisciplinary approach to spiritual care is put forward, whilst acknowledging that nurses, as primary carers, have a central role as enablers in empowering patients to achieve spiritual growth. The emerging debates about some of the problems connected to establishing spirituality as a concept in health care were examined and there appears to be a lack of consensus about what spirituality and spiritual care are. In spite of the various diverse perspectives on spirituality, several authors appear to converge on the point that spirituality is an important facet of humanity, and attention to this dimension is central to health care. If nurses and health carers ignore patients' spirituality, then they are denying part of their very existence.

References

Aldridge, A. (2003) *Consumption*. Polity, Cambridge.

Aldridge, D. (2000) *Spirituality, Healing and Medicine*. Jessica Kingsley, London.

Baldacchino, D. (2003) *Spirituality in Illness and Care*. Price Library, Malta.

Baldacchino, D. and Draper, P. (2001) Spiritual coping strategies: A review of the nursing research literature. *Journal of Advanced Nursing*, **34**(6), 833–41.

Benson, H. and Stark, M. (1996) *Timeless Healing: Power and Biology of Belief*. Simon & Schuster, London.

Bowie, R. (2001) *Ethical Studies*. Nelson Thomas, Cheltenham.

Brierley, P. (ed.) (2000) *Religious Trends 2000*. HarperCollins, London.

Bradshaw, A. (1994) *Lighting the Lamp: The Spiritual Dimension of Nursing Care*. Scutari Press, London.

Bruce, E. (1998) How can we measure spiritual well-being? *Journal of Dementia*, May/June, 16–17.

Burr, V. (2003) *Social Constructionism*, 2nd edn. Routledge, London.

Butler, C. (2002) *Postmodernism*. Oxford University Press, Oxford.

Catterall, R. A., Cox, M., Greet, B., Sankey, J. and Griffiths, G. (1998) The assessment and audit of spiritual care. *International Journal of Palliative Nursing*, **4**(4), 162–8.

Chopra, D. (1989) *Quantum Healing; Exploring the Frontiers of Mind/Body Medicine*. Bantam Books, New York.

Chopra, D. (2000) *How to Know God. The Soul's Journey Into the Mystery of Mysteries*. Rider, London.

Clark, C. C., Cross, J. R., Deane, D. M. and Lowery, L. W. (1991) Spirituality: integral to quality care. *Holistic Nursing Practice*, **5**(3), 67–76.

Coyle, J. (2002) Spirituality and health: towards a framework for exploring the relationship between spirituality and health. *Journal of Advanced Nursing*, **37**(6), 589–97.

Dossey, L. (1993) *Healing Words: the Power of Prayer and the Practice of Medicine*. Harper, San Francisco.

Draper, P. and McSherry, W. (2002) A critical view of spirituality and spiritual assessment. *Journal of Advanced Nursing*, **39**, 1–2.

Dunniece, U. and Slevin, E. (2000) Nurses' experience of being present with a patient receiving a diagnosis of cancer. *Journal of Advanced Nursing*, **32**(3), 611–18.

Farran, C. J., Fitchett, G., Quiring-Emlen, J. D. and Burck, J. R. (1989) Development of a model of spiritual assessment and intervention. *Journal of Religion and Health*, **28**(3), 185–95.

Fellow, W. (1978) *Religions: East and West*. Holt, Rinehart and Winston, New York.

Frankl, V. E. (1967) *Man's Search for Meaning*. Washington Square Press, New York.

Fry, E. (1997) Spirituality: connectedness through being and doing. In: *Spirituality: The Heart of Nursing* (ed. S. Ronaldson). Alismed Publications, Melbourne.

Goldberg, B. (1998) Connection: an exploration of spirituality in nursing care. *Journal of Advanced Nursing*, **27**, 836–42.

Govier, I. (2000) Spiritual care in nursing: a systematic approach. *Nursing Standard*, **14**(17), 32–6.

Haase, J. E. (1987) Components of courage in chronically ill adolescents: a phenomenological study. *Advanced Nursing Science*, **9**(2), 64–80.

Hardy A. (1987) *The Spiritual Nature of Man*. Oxford University Press, Oxford.

Hay, D. (1987) *Exploring Inner Space*. Mowbray, London.

Henery, N. (2003) Constructions of spirituality in contemporary nursing theory. *Journal of Advanced Nursing*, **42**(6), 550–7.

Henley, A. and Schott, J. (1999) *Culture, Religion and Patient Care in Multiethnic Society*. Age Concern, London.

Highfields, M. F. and Cason, C. (1993) Spiritual needs of patients: are they recognised? *Cancer Nursing*, June, 187–92.

Holland, K. and Hogg, C. (2001) *Cultural Awareness in Nursing and Health Care: An Introductory Text*. Arnold, London.

Jacik, M. (1986) Personal communcation. In *Spiritual Dimensions of Nursing Practice* (ed. V. B. Carson). W. B. Saunders, Philadelphia.

James, W. (1983) *The Varieties of Religious Experience*. Penguin, London.

Kim, M. J., McFarland, S. K. and McLane, A. M. (1984) *Pocket Guide to Nursing Diagnosis*. Mosby, St Louis.

Kissane, C. (2004) Spiritual nursing care of older adults. *Nurse 2 Nurse*, **4**(4), 29–32.

Koenig, H. (2000) Religion, spirituality, and medicine: application to clinical practice. *Journal of the American Medical Association*, **284**(13), 1708.

Koenig, H. G. (2001) *Spirituality in Patient Care: Why, How, When and What?* Templeton Foundation Press, Radnor, Pennsylvania.

Koenig, H. G. (2002) An 83-year old woman with chronic illness and strong religious health. *Journal of the American Medical Association*, **288**, 487–93.

Kuhn, C. C. (1988) A spiritual inventory of the medical ill patients. *Psychiatric Medicine*, **6**, 87–100.

Larson, D. B., Sherrill, K. A., Lyons, J. S., Craigie, F. C., Thielman, S. B., Greenwood, M. A. and Larson, S. S. (1992) Associations between dimensions of religious commitment and mental health reported in the *American Journal of Mental Health and Archives of General Psychiatry*: 1078–1989. *American Journal of Psychiatry*, **149**(4), 557–9.

Larson, D. B., Swyers, J. P. and McCullough, M. (1998) *Scientific Research on Spirituality and Health: a Consensus Report*. National Institute of Healthcare Research, Rockville, Maryland.

Lazarus, R. S. and Folkman, S. (1984). *Stress, Appraisal and Coping*. Springer, New York.

Linbeck, G. A. (1984) *The Nature of Doctrine*. Westminster Press, Philadelphia.

Macaskill, A. (2002) *Heal the Hurt. How to Forgive and Move On.* Sheldon Press, London.

MacLaren, J. (2004) A kaleidoscope of understandings: spiritual nursing in a multi-faith society. *Journal of Advanced Nursing*, **45**(5), 457–64.

MacKinlay, E. (2001) *The Spiritual Dimensions of Ageing.* Jessica Kingsley, London.

Maugan, T. A. (1996) The SPIRITual history. *Archives of Family Medicine*, **5**(1), 11–16.

Maslow, A. R. (1968) *Towards a Psychology of Being.* Van Nostrand, New York.

Matthews, D. A. (1998) *The Faith Factor: Proof of the Healing Power of Prayer.* Penguin Books, New York.

McSherry, W. (2000) *Making Sense of Spirituality in Nursing Practice.* Churchill Livingstone, Edinburgh.

McSherry, W. and Watson, R. (2002) Spirituality in nursing care: evidence of a gap between theory and practice. *Journal of Clinical Nursing*, **11**, 843–4.

McSherry, W. and Ross, L. (2002) Dilemmas of spiritual assessment; considerations for nursing practice. *Journal of Advanced Nursing*, **38**(5), 478–88.

MORI (2003) *Three in Five 'Believe in God'.* http://www.mori.co.uk/polls/2003/bbc-heavenandearth.shtml.

Murray, R. and Zentner, J. B. (1989) *Nursing Concepts for Health Promotion.* Prentice Hall, London.

Narayanasamy, A. (2001) *Spiritual Care: A Practical Guide for Nurses and Health Care Practitioners*, 2nd edn. Quay, Wiltshire.

Narayanasamy, A. (2002) Spiritual coping mechanisms in chronically ill patients. *British Journal of Nursing*, **11**, 1461–70.

Narayanasamy, A. (2004) The puzzle of spirituality for nursing: a guide to practical assessment. *British Journal of Nursing*, **13**(19), 1140–4.

Narayanasamy, A. and Andrews, A. (2000) Cultural impact of Islam on the future directions of nursing education. *Nurse Education Today*, **7**(1), 57–64.

Narayanasamy, A. and Owen, J. (2001) A critical incident study of nurses' responses to the spiritual needs of their patients. *Journal of Advanced Nursing*, **33**(4), 446–55.

Narayanasamy, A., Gates, B. and Swinton, J. (2002) Spirituality and learning disabilities: a qualitative study. *British Journal of Nursing*, **11**(14), 948–51.

Newberg, A., D'Aquili, E. and Rause, V. (2002) *Why God Won't Go Away: Brain Science and the Biology of Belief.* Ballantine Books, New York.

O'Brien, M. E. (1982) Religious faith and adjustment to long-term haemodialysis. *Journal of Religious Health*, **21**, 68.

O'Brien, M. E. (2003) *Spirituality in Nursing*, 2nd edn. Jones & Bartlett, London.

Otto, R. (1950) *The Idea of the Holy* (transl. John W. Harvey). Oxford University Press, Oxford.

Parfitt, B. (1998) *Working Across Cultures: A Study of Expatriate Nurses Working in Developing Countries in Primary Health Care*. Ashage, Aldershot.

Parrinder, G. (1968) *Asian Religions*. Sheldon Press, London.

Post, S. and Puchalski, C. (2000) Physicians and patient spirituality: professional boundaries, competency, and ethics. *Annals of Internal Medicine*, **132**(7), 578–83.

Roach, M. (1991) The call to consciousness: compassion in today's health world. In: *In Caring: The Compassionate Healer* (eds. L. Gaul and M. Leininger), pp. 7–18. National League for Nursing, New York.

Ross, L. (1997) *Nurses' Perceptions of Spiritual Care*. Avebury, Aldershot.

Ross, L. (1998) The nurses role in spiritual care. In *The Spiritual Challenge of Health Care* (eds. M. Cobb and V. Robshaw). Churchill Livingstone, Edinburgh.

Rousseau, P. (2000) Spirituality and the dying patient. *Journal of Clinical Oncology*, **18**(9), 2000–2.

Scott Littleton, C. (1996) *The Sacred East*. Duncan Baird, London.

Shelly, J. A. (2000) *Spiritual Care: A Guide for Caregivers*. InterVarsity Press.

Shelley, A. L. and Fish, S. (1988) *Spiritual Care: The Nurse's Role*. Inter Varsity Press, Illinois.

Sherwood, G. D. (2000) The power of nurse–client encounters. *Journal of Holistic Nursing*, **18**(2), 159–75.

Stoll, R. G. (1979) Guidelines for spiritual assessment. *American Journal of Nursing*, **79**, 1574–7.

Stolley, J. M. and Koenig, H. (1997) Religion/spirituality and health among elderly African Americans and Hispanics. *Journal of Psychosocial Nursing and Mental Health Services*, **35**, 32–8.

Swinton, J. (2001) *Spirituality and Mental Health Care*. Jessica Kingsley, London.

Swinton, J. and Narayanasamy, A. (2002) Jan Forum: Response to 'A critical view of spirituality and spiritual assessment' by P. Draper and W. McSherry (2002) *Journal of Advanced Nursing*, **39**, 1–2. *Journal of Advanced Nursing*, **40**(2), 158–60.

Thomsen, R. (1998) Spirituality in medical practice. *Archives Dematology*, **134**(11), 1443–6.

Warren, R. (2002) *The Purpose Driven Life*. Zondervan, Michigan.

Wallis, R. (1984) *The Elementary Forms of New Religious Life*. Routledge, London.

Woods, T. (1999) *Beginning Postmodernism*. Manchester University Press, Manchester and New York.

CHAPTER 3

Transcultural health care

Aru Narayanasamy and Ethelrene White

Summary

This chapter provides a review of transcultural health care in the light of the literature and developments in the context of Britain. In so doing, the key features of transcultural nursing are explored and commented on in terms of the following: definitions, racism, ethnocentrism, culture, diversity, transcultural health care practice, legislation and reports, transcultural health care nurse education and models of practice. There is promising evidence from emerging literature that innovations are taking place in promoting transcultural care practice and education. However, the conclusions drawn in this chapter are that much practice-based research is still needed to establish transcultural nursing in Britain.

Key points:

- Approaches to transcultural health care are gaining momentum in the UK.
- The impact of globalisation, diversity, culture, ethnicity and identity is felt in the health care setting, making transcultural health care relevant.
- Transcultural health care should be an important part of the nurse education curriculum.
- The ACCESS Model offers a framework for transcultural health care education.

Introduction

Many people from minority ethnic communities in Britain, have different cultural needs and belief systems than those of the indigenous population (Narayanasamy, 2002). Some of these people require health care that is cognisant of their diverse cultural needs (Ahmad, 1993; Cortis, 1993; Thomas and Dines, 1994; Rassool, 1995; Fletcher, 1997; Duffy, 2001; Holland and Hogg, 2001). Various National Health Service (NHS) initiatives in the UK emphasise patients and communities as being central to the provision of services (Cortis, 2003; Foolchand, 2000). For example, the NHS Plan (Department of Health, 2000) and the National Service Framework (NSF) (Chady, 2001; Foolchand, 2000) highlight that services should be responsive to individuals and communities, including attention to the cultural aspects of people's lives. Nurse educational initiatives in Britain include the *Benchmark Statement: Health Care Programmes*, which specifies attention to cultural needs (Quality Assurance Agency for Higher Education, 2001). Likewise, there is a proliferation of transcultural health care literature signalling the importance of cultural competence in the USA, Canada, New Zealand and Australia (Anderson *et al.*, 2003; Duffy, 2001; Eisenbruch, 2001; Polachek, 1998).

However, there is growing concern that the cultural health care needs of minority ethnic groups are not met adequately (Ahmad, 1993; Thomas and Dines, 1994; Rassool, 1995; Gerrish *et al.*, 1996; Fletcher, 1997; Papadopoulos *et al.*, 1998; Le Var, 1998; Gerrish and Papadopoulos, 1999; Foolchand, 2000; Duffy 2001; Serrant Green, 2001; Nairn *et al.*, 2004). There is a litany of evidence to suggest the failures of measures to improve provisions to meet the health, social and educational needs of people from minority ethnic groups in the UK. This includes failures of multicultural education, structures and policies, and transcultural health care practices (Gerrish *et al.*, 1996). There is the suggestion that a fuller commitment to implement transcultural health care practices based on research will eradicate the existing anomalies in the health care provisions for people from the minority ethnic groups (Narayanasamy, 2002).

Definition of transcultural health care

Transcultural health care is defined by Leininger (1997a) as:

> formal areas of study and practice in the cultural beliefs, values and lifeways of diverse cultures and in the use of knowledge to provide culture-specific or culture-universal care to individuals, families and groups of particular cultures.

Herberg (1989) believes that nursing care provided 'in a manner that is sensitive to the needs of individuals, families and groups who represent diverse cultural population within a society' is transcultural nursing.

Globalisation, culture, ethnicity and identity

Before pursuing the merits of transcultural nursing, it should first be established what culture is. Culture affects virtually every aspect of daily life – how we think, behave, and make judgements and decisions. Put simply, culture can be defined as 'how we do and view things in our group' (Henley and Schott, 1999). Hofstede (1991) views culture as being acquired unconsciously in early childhood. Most people, especially those who are members of the majority culture, grow up unaware that they have a specific culture. They may not realise that what they perceive as normal, universal values and ways of behaving are in fact cultural, and 'normal' only to their group or social class. On the other hand, people who have grown up as members of a minority ethnic group, or who have lived outside or away from their own society, are acutely aware of culture and its influence. Sometimes, they may even jettison their own culture in an attempt to 'fit in', whilst others go through the acculturation process by acquiring dominant cultural values. However, postmodernists such as Modood (1992) note that the globalisation of culture has led to national cultural identities being eroded. British culture is not immune, and all ethnicities, including white, have begun to 'pick and mix', with emerging new hybrid identities. Racial and ethnic differences become a matter of choice, making it difficult to discuss racial disadvantage, as ethnic identity is not fixed.

Globalisation

Many western and eastern countries' economies, health and education depend on international investment and cooperation which appears to be tolerant of ethnic and cultural influences in terms of consumerism. In other words, globalisation and international trade agreements are advantageous to the Western world, and therefore other ethnicities are tolerated for the sake of economic interests. The national and local economies and livelihoods may be totally dependent upon foreign money. However, in many instances when it comes to equality and respect for humanity at an individual level, attitudes of ambivalence prevail in terms of skin colour, ethnicity, social class and religion. For some, the oppression of vulnerable minority groups is the means to maintaining power and status by dominant cultural groups (Parfitt, 1998). Any threats to these power relations are thwarted by oppressive discriminatory practices, which may be overt or covert.

Furthermore, globalisation is seen to pervade nationhood and cultural identities (Guibernau and Goldblatt, 2000). There is a concern that Britain is being taken over by an invasion of other cultures, religions, norms and values. In response to this, there is a call for the preservation of British identity and culture by raising the profile of Britishness and its culture. In Britain the view of the extreme right is that, this nation cannot and should not accept black ethnic minorities, and it vociferously advocates repatriation. According to Guibernau and Goldblatt, there are signs that a new sense of 'Britishness' is slowly emerging in the field of popular culture, especially in the worlds of food, fashion and music. This revival of Britishness has been shaped by the traditional but also, ironically, by multiculturalism and globalisation.

Others argue that the views of the extreme right are unacceptable and call for the full integration of ethnic minorities into the dominant host culture. However, it is less clear what constitutes full integration. Moreover, when some individuals from black minority ethnic groups attempted to integrate by acquiring the language, educational and professional qualifications, values and beliefs of the dominant culture they found that opportunities for social and economic advancement by occupational mobility were blocked, as many of the dominant population were frequently hostile because of their consciously held and subliminal racist attitudes (Narayanasamy, 1999a; Wright, 1991). Some others view integration to mean a pluralistic society, a milieu in which minority ethnic people exercise autonomy in their cultural beliefs and practices whilst conforming to the demands of law and order.

Guibernau and Goldblatt (2000) are optimistic that multiculturalism and diversity will flourish in the UK, although they are realistic enough to acknowledge that racism and British imperial history may act as obstacles. They highlight that the process of acquiring an English or British identity may mean stereotyping and labelling minorities so that they can be discriminated against. Institutional racism may prove to be an even greater obstacle to equal opportunities. Likewise, there is likely to be a rise in affluent white middle class gated communities to ensure the exclusion not only of the less well-off members of society but of minority ethnic groups as well.

Cultures are maps of meaning in which the world is made intelligible. Cultural diversity and differences are hailed as the panacea for providing a culturally sensitive approach to the care of minority ethic groups. Leininger (1997a) is acknowledged as the pioneer of transcultural nursing. Leininger brought an anthropological perspective to the care of people from minority ethnic backgrounds. According to the literature, four perspectives prevail with regard to cultural care in the context of health care. These are assimilation and multiculturalism; a culturalist approach; an anti-racist approach; and a pluralistic approach. Each one of these has strengths and weaknesses. What follows is a critical examination of each of these approaches in the context of the literature.

Assimilation and multiculturalism

Multiculturalism was at its height in the 1960s and 1970s, when social, educational and economic policies were put in place in the UK to promote the integration and assimilation of immigrant communities into the main society (Gerrish *et al.*, 1996; Narayanasamy, 1999a). Multiculturalism aimed to promote policies designed to support minority ethnic communities to engage in the learning of the language and culture of the host society. It was envisioned then that such policies would make the process of integration and assimilation easier. This strategy was seen as a means to enhance race relations and that the dominant white society would be tolerant of new arrivals who are willing to adapt and assimilate into the British way of life. Adaptation and assimilation were seen as possible through being proficient in the language and customs of Britain. Equally, it was perceived as the ideal by policymakers and some people from the minority ethnic communities. They saw multiculturalism as an avenue that promised to open up opportunities for newly arrived immigrants to become part of the dominant culture and gain full membership of the society by enjoying the rights and full trappings of the main society.

However, according to Gerrish *et al.* (1996) and Narayanasamy (1999b), multiculturalism was far from being a success for a number of reasons. When minority ethnic groups attempted to acquire the language and culture of the dominant cultural group they found many barriers to opportunities with regard to employment, housing and education. Obstacles were stacked against them in terms of racial discrimination and hostility, social exclusion and isolation. Apart from barriers to jobs, education and welfare rights, many faced problems of full access to health care and treatment as well. Substantial evidence comes from the literature with regard to such barriers (Ahmad, 1983; Fernando, 1991; Gerrish *et al.*, 1996; Gerrish and Papadapoulos, 1999; Narayanasamy, 1999b). It is worth noting that the New Labour government appears to be supportive of the need for minority ethnic communities to be proficient in English. Although the intentions of the government may be right, this is seen as soft racism to please right-wing Labour supporters. In response to the failures of assimilation and multiculturalism, the culturalist approach explored in the next section was advocated. The culturalist approach is largely based on the premise that an enlightened dominant population with a sound understanding of cultural diversity and meanings would be more receptive and tolerant of people of other cultures.

Culturalist approach

The culturalist approach, based on the work of Leininger (1997a), was promoted as the ideal model of a culturally sensitive approach. Such an approach
was based on the premise that if greater awareness of minority cultures was
created, there would be better understanding about people who are different in terms of racial identity, ethnicity and culture. It was speculated that
this would lead to harmonious mutual exchanges and understanding between
groups. Such awareness would, it was believed, lead to the removal of prejudices and stereotypes that arise out of ignorance and misguided perceptions.
However, the culturalist approach as espoused by Leininger came under criticism on the grounds that it reinforces cultural stereotypes by sensationalising
cultures as exotic products. It is also accused of ignoring the issue of racism.
Critics believed that oppression and discrimination were rooted in racism, in
part due to the legacies of western colonialism, imperialism and dominance.
Therefore an anti-racist approach was put forward as an alternative to the
culturalist approach.

Anti-racist perspective

The anti-racist perspective is that the evils of racism should be acknowledged and rooted out. Anti-racist writers argue that racism is prevalent in all
western societies in the form of personal and institutional racism. Equally,
the right-wing media, educational and social policies, power and status are
blamed for oppression. Racists exert their power over vulnerable groups
such as minority ethnic people and subject them to harassment and discrimination by overt and covert measures. Personal racism may be subtle
and hidden within structures which may manifest as institutional racism.
Institutional racism received much attention as a result of the inquiry into
the death of a black teenager, Stephen Lawrence (Macpherson, 1999). The
Macpherson Report was critical of the police for institutional racism and
attributed this to their failure to bring a successful prosecution against the
alleged murderers of the black teenager.

Institutional racism

The Macpherson Report reaffirmed the phrase 'institutional racism', which is
prevalent in most of Britain's public institutions. For the purpose of its inquiry,
institutional racism is defined (Macpherson, 1999, p. 10) as:

The collective failure of an organisation to provide an appropriate and professional service to people because of their colour, culture, or ethnic origin. It
can be seen or detected in processes, attitudes and behaviour which amount
to discrimination through unwitting prejudice, ignorance, thoughtlessness
and racist stereotyping which disadvantage minority ethnic people.

There is evidence that institutional racism pervades health care, including
nursing (Sawley, 2001). This may be one possible reason for the slow pace
in the development of culturally sensitive care and responsiveness to cultural
diversity initiatives. Anderson *et al.* (2003, p. 207) suggest that 'race, class,
culture and gender may unwittingly be a subtext, for deciding who needs help,
who does not, and what the priorities are at any given moment in time'. Sawley
(2001) acknowledges that institutional racism in not a new phenomenon but is
evident in many areas of government responsibility, such as local government,
housing, social work, employment, education policy and politics.

According to the anti-racist perspective, the only way to eradicate oppression
and injustice to minority ethnic groups is by addressing racism at the personal
and institutional levels. Anti-discriminatory practices are moral imperatives that
must be introduced and implemented wholeheartedly. It is the hallmark of a just
and civilised society that active measures are put in place at all levels to eradicate racism and oppression of all vulnerable groups.

However, in spite of the moral arguments of the anti-racist perspective it
draws criticisms. It accuses white people of being racists, and is also discriminatory in reverse because it appears to tarnish all people with the same brush.
It is offensive to well-intended white people who want a just society as well.
The anti-racist perspective is retrospective, blaming and uncompromising in that
some people are made to feel guilty about past events: historical racist acts committed by ancestors. It is almost dismissive of the emerging measures and good
practices related to cultural diversity and differences. However, the pluralistic
approach appears to offer a promising alternative to the anti-racist approach.

Pluralistic approach

The pluralistic approach appears to align with postmodernism in acknowledging
the multicultural and multiethnic nature of a society. It attempts to reconcile the
best elements of the above three approaches. It emphasises cultural pluralism
and attempts to respond to cultural differences. The pluralists seek to find measures to establish connections between communities by celebrating the richness
of cultural diversity and differences. The Department of Health has put in place
many strategic policies to implement cultural diversity programmes and to promote connections by openly recognising the value of diversity to the nation and

its economy. However, in spite of its good intentions, the pluralistic approach is criticised for underplaying the issue of racism and being too compromising by ignoring oppression. In spite of this criticism, the pluralistic approach offers a way forward in promoting good practices in society and health care services to improve the quality of life for people from minority ethnic backgrounds.

Transcultural health care practice

The previous statutory professional body, the English National Board (ENB) instituted a number of initiatives to improve education related to transcultural health care practices. Within its statutory responsibilities in relation to education provision for pre- and post-registration education, the English National Board for Nursing, Midwifery and Health Visiting acknowledged the need for nurses to be prepared to meet effectively the health care needs of minority ethnic groups. This requirement is explicit within the Nurses, Midwives and Health Visitors Act 1989 (Rule 18a) relating to the implementation of Project 2000 and in the more recent developments in nurse education (ENB, 2000; UKCC, 1999). The ENB incorporated a policy for equal opportunities and anti-racism in the Regulations and Guidelines for the approval of courses and institutions. To reflect increasing pluralism within society, this policy emphasised the need for a more holistic approach in clinical practice. Moreover, the ENB recognised the importance of education in explaining cultural, family and economic influences in the prevention of ill health and disease (ENB, 1993). This approach was augmented in the document *Standards for the Approval of Higher Education Institutions and Programmes* (ENB, 1997).

The National Health Service initiated major policies to address the promotion of transcultural competence in health care, and the promotion of equal opportunities (NHSE, 1999). The ENB commissioned three projects which investigated whether nurses and midwives were adequately prepared to meet the health care needs of ethnic groups. The first report was published by Gerrish *et al.* (1996), and provided recommendations for health care professionals in acquiring and developing multi/transcultural competencies.

Multicultural Britain

The literature acknowledges that Britain is regarded as one of the most ethnically diverse countries in Europe (Ahmad, 1993; Baxter, 2000; Rassool, 1995; Gerrish *et al.*, 1996; Peberdy, 1997; Le Var, 1998). According to the 2001 population census, about 9% of people in England claimed to belong to Black and other minority ethnic (BME) groups. Thus it is within this ethnically diverse society that health care providers must deliver a service that is culturally sensitive and appropriate to meet specific needs (Narayanasamy, 2002).

From a historical perspective, the NHS can be perceived as a service created to meet the health care needs of the British people (Cortis, 1993). Its provision evolved naturally around British social and family patterns, embracing religious and cultural beliefs (Wilkins, 1993). It responded predominantly to the expectations and health needs of the indigenous population at that time. According to Parfitt (1998, p. 50), the health service 'reflects the cultural norm of not only the white majority but the middle class white majority'. It perpetuated the belief that the 'white' person is the norm and not only black people but also those who are disadvantaged, deprived and underprivileged were considered to be different. Such perspectives are seen as preventing 'health providers from forming normal relationships with black clients' (Parfitt, 1998, p. 50).

According to Narayanasamy (2002), 'push and pull factors' prompted the migration of people of diverse ethnicities, cultures, religions and spiritualities to Britain. According to Papadopoulos *et al.* (1998, p. 49), 'Throughout the 19th and into the 20th Century the colonies continued to make their own contribution to the British economy, their men fought in both wars while their native economies were systematically underdeveloped'. Economic deprivation acted as the push factors in compelling people from the Caribbean and the Asian subcontinent to succumb to the persuasion and propaganda of recruiters in the 1950s and 1960s. The promise of a bright future and the desire for economic improvement in Britain were strong pull factors that attracted not only the unemployed but also some who held skilled and secure jobs (Papadopoulos *et al.*, 1998). More recently, Britain has attracted refugees from the East and West for reasons of political oppression, ethnic cleansing, civil war and natural disasters. Apart from this, there is a transient population of international status who reside here as students, business people and others on exchange visits. All universities in the UK attract students and academics from the international communities, all bringing diverse ethnic and cultural influences that enrich, enliven and prevent fossilisation of British culture. Moreover, previously economically depressed cities such as Leicester, contrary to fears about the impact of settlers from the immigrant communities, actually benefited following the wealth creation that resulted from the presence of Asians from East Africa.

Dominant values

It has been suggested that the majority of nursing is delivered from the value position of carers which may be based on their dominant cultural beliefs

(Stokes, 1991). Ironically, the vast majority of indigenous health care workers have rarely, if ever, previously given consideration as to what their values and cultural beliefs are, or how their values, beliefs and cultural traditions are acquired. Yet most assume, with equal measures of ignorance and arrogance, that their 'British' culture is the right way and that it is naturally superior to all other 'uncivilised or unsophisticated' cultures. Regrettably, such an approach may be antagonistic and unhelpful to patients/clients who are not Anglicised or British. That negative tension or cultural conflict, if not rapidly dispelled, will ultimately undermine the therapeutic relationship between patient and carer; and therefore the quality of care will be compromised.

The process of occupational socialisation in nursing, exposes students and nurses to adapt and internalise the values of the dominant culture. Therefore nursing is embedded in a specific culture that pervades all aspects of care and practice. In this context, nursing is not culturally free but culturally determined, and if this is not acknowledged or understood then nurses are in danger of being guilty of gross ethnocentrism (Stokes, 1991). According to Parfitt (1998, p. 52):

> Nurses who hold ethnocentric views will be unable to interpret their patients' behaviour appropriately as they will judge it according to norms of their own behaviour.

Research, knowledge and competence

A transcultural health care approach based on research knowledge and competence offers a basis for how to care for people who, due to their cultural needs, require sensitive consideration (Macdonald, 1987; Littlewood and Lipsedge, 1981; Rothenburger, 1990; McGee, 1992; Rassool, 1995; Gerrish *et al.*, 1996). The sparse literature on nurse education seeks more guidance and direction on how transcultural care is planned, delivered and implemented, rather than coming up with its own suggestions (Rassool, 1994; Gerrish *et al.*, 1996; Fletcher, 1997). From the perspectives of health care users (minority ethnic communities), educators, practitioners and students; Gerrish and colleagues (1996) make recommendations for transcultural health care education. They propose a model for transcultural health care practice which incorporates the development of cultural sensitivity (the practitioner as a tourist), reflexive honesty, re-examination of ethnicity, intercultural communication and associated stress, measures to eradicate racism (particularly institutional), concerted efforts to improve policies and procedures related to recruitment, and selection of candidates from ethnic communities. In addition to this model, the planning and delivery of transcultural health care programmes can be effective if specific learning materials are available (Narayanasamy, 1998).

Much of the literature on transcultural health care is written in the context of North American populations (Leininger, 1997a), although the emerging literature in the UK offers some useful theoretical perspectives in the context of multicultural Britain (Dobson, 1991; Stokes, 1991; McGee, 1992; Cortis, 1993; Wilkins, 1993; Thomas and Dines, 1994; Gerrish *et al.*, 1996; Le Var, 1998; Gerrish and Papadopoulos, 1999; Parfitt, 1998; Narayanasamy, 1999a,b, 2002, 2003; Holland and Hogg, 2001). The literature describes the following as desirable for the implementation of transcultural health care practices. An extensive database of health care information about culturally determined aspects of health, illness and care may help to improve transcultural care. This can be enhanced by the provision of culture-specific and culture-sensitive nursing care (Macdonald, 1987; Leininger, 1997a), but at the same time placing an emphasis on caring acts as universal but taking many forms and variations in many cultures (Leininger, 1997b). This approach can be further strengthened if health care practitioners consider that systems of treatment and care may already prevail in other cultures and integrate these into current practice (Dobson, 1991). In regard to this, Leininger (1997b) stresses that attention should be paid to the significance of 'folk systems' and these need to be incorporated into professional approaches to care. However, Gerrish *et al.* (1996) caution that without opportunities for self-awareness development (subjecting self to challenges of assumptions), health care practitioners are less likely to show sensitivity to other cultural values. In a similar vein, Baxter (2000) warns that one's own values, if imposed on others, can be offensive and unprofessional. In such circumstances clients may actually avoid carers.

However, this literature lacks systematic evaluation (Gerrish *et al.*, 1996), and the rhetoric on transcultural health care lacks guidance on practical implementation (Ahmad, 1993). Furthermore, due to policies imposed by the ENB (1993) and UKCC (1999), and health care legislation (Gerrish *et al.*, 1996), nurses and other health care practitioners may feel under pressure to implement transcultural health care haphazardly. Yet without the necessary education, training and learning material it may compound some of the problems, as identified in the literature (Bruni, 1988; Kerslake, 1988; Friedman, 1990; Rothenburger, 1991; Baxter, 2000).

Leininger's theory of transcultural care

Five decades have elapsed since Leininger first recognised the importance of understanding the significance of other ethnicities' cultural lifeways based on their value and belief systems. So full of conviction was Leininger regarding the pivotal importance of this fundamental specialist knowledge to the effective

DoH policies implement cultural
diversity programmes.

English National Board:

→ Britain: most ethnically diverse
countries in Europe

Historically: NHS meant for middle, upper
class white people.

Castles & Miller 02 'push + pull facks'

refugees from East + west → political oppression,
ethnic cleansing, civil war + natural disasks.
→ students, business, exchange visits.

eg Hitch (1998 p52): Nurses who hold
ethnocentric views will be unable to interpret
their patients' behaviour appropriately as they
will judge it according to norms of their
own.

3000

stats policy literature.

300 Intro.

Background.

1200 → Current Research → rationale for st
& aims + objectives.   ?

1200 → Methodology, method, ethics.
narrative.   timetable.   ?

300 Conclusion.

• Most assume British culture is the right way
  – no consideration how acquired.
  – unhelpful

Table 3.1 Legislation and reports which act as drivers of change.

- Sir Donald Acheson's Report (1998) *The Independent Inquiry into Inequalities in Health*
- The Human Rights Act (1998)
- Sir William Macpherson's Report (1999) The Stephen Lawrence Inquiry
- Department of Health (1999) Saving Lives: Our Healthier Nation. HMSO: London
- Ziggi Alexander (2000) Study of Black, Asian and Ethnic Minority Issues; Department of Health: London
- European Convention on Human Rights (enacted 2 October 2000)
- The Race Relations (Amendment) Act (2000) (enacted 31 May 2002)

practice of nursing that she embarked on a lengthy period of ethnographic study, resulting in the production of approximately 100 culture-specific studies.

There is now a body of knowledge that professional nursing can access, if it so wishes. Leininger (1997a,b) held the view that care was powerful in healing and that there could be no curing without caring. Thus, she 'gave birth' to the concept of transcultural nursing, the goal of which is to provide culturally congruent care that is tailored to cultural specific care values and lifeways.

It was Leininger's hope that the research-based evidence generated by her culture care theory would provide knowledge to support the discipline of transcultural nursing. Leininger's vision is that by the year 2020, transcultural care will have transcended all aspects of nursing globally (Leininger, 2001). However, critics point out that Leininger's model is a passive statement of good intent which is based on free will and the assumption that all good nurses want to provide culturally specific care. Her model fails to address the real 'heart of the matter'; the issues of prejudice and racism (Eisenbruch, 2001; Narayanasamy, 1999a). Here in the UK it is most likely that the pieces of legislation listed in Table 3.1 will force the changes to come about. Further criticisms of Leininger's theory of transcultural care are explored in the next section.

Criticisms of transcultural care

A further criticism of Leininger's work is that in romanticising non-white cultures she overlooks racism. There could have been an explicit critique of racism and Western etic perspectives of other cultures. Leininger's work is largely based on ethnography and perhaps there is a need to incorporate feminist poststructural and post-colonial discourses to examine culture as a notion. Postcolonial discourses scholars such as Gandhi (1998) and Gilroy (2000) call for a critical review of the concept of culture (Anderson *et al.*, 2003). They argue that like 'race', culture is socially constructed and is laden with social, political and historical meanings. Post-colonial and post-national feminists call for a re-examination of such an approach to cultural care in nursing by shifting the focus away from the preoccupation with exotic belief system of people from different ethnocultural backgrounds, and regarding each group as distinctive entity (Anderson *et al.*, 2003). In this sense, Leininger's transcultural nursing takes an essentialist approach in presenting culture as fixed and peculiar to particular ethnic groups. Instead, health care practitioners should examine the unequal relations of power as a consequence of the colonial past and neo-colonial present as well as the prevailing ideologies that have redefined local meanings and dictated social structures, including the health care delivery systems. In other words, the focus should be on the Western medical framework and its culture and ideologies, which have constructed health care discourses whilst silencing other voices.

According to Culley (2001), Qureshi (1989) and Rack (1990) have been instrumental in producing distorted notions of cultural cohesive communities in the UK. These notions of cultural communities were portrayed with negative stereotypes. Qureshi and Rack use the biomedical discourse in perpetuating the essentialist view of ethnicity and culture. Such a misguided approach is limiting in homogenising and perpetuating stereotypical versions of cultural beliefs and practices of the socially constructed 'other'. Cultures framed in rigid and static terms are regarded as British or 'aliens'. People are treated as the other or British usually in terms of whiteness or physical characteristics such as skin colour, culture, religion and so on. Diversity and differences are redefined and reproduced by social construction and presented as the 'other'. According to Culley (2001, p. 111), people are stereotyped using culturalist's framework:

'West Indians' for example, are stereotypically described as resentful of authority, having low educational standards and being involved in drugs and crime. Asian families are seen as close-knit and industrious but very different culturally. In recent years Muslims in particular have been characterised as aliens and intolerant fanatics who pose a threat to the 'British way of life'

In reality, individuals renegotiate, intersect, transact, compromise and adapt throughout their life course and trajectories of illness, structural barriers and social divisions. However, in defence of the culturalist's approach, it brings into focus the importance of cultural sensitivity in nursing and health care practices. In spite of its colonial legacy and anthropological traditions, transcultural perspectives have an enduring hold on nursing by offering an apparent framework for responding with sensitivity to the cultural, spiritual and religious needs of patients and clients. Culturalists claim to take an inclusive approach to the cultural needs of patient in a multi-ethnic and multicultural context of health care. However, Gunaratnam (1997) criticises that in doing so, cultural-ists have created factfiles on cultural beliefs and practices which are unhelpful. Such an approach ignores diversity and the individual's agency for negotiat-ing, or simply for being a human requiring holistic understanding rather than a socially constructed person with imagined attributes and categories as the 'other'. Gunaratnam (1997) argues that factfiles reinforce a myopic view of culture as one-dimensional, 'frozen in time and context' (Culley, 2001, p. 122). The culturalist focus leads to packaging cultural practices with patients' choices, and this precedence sidelines or ignores their need for holistic care, including emotional support. The reductionist approach to multicultural practices renders professional interaction as highly task-orientated. Until a consensus is reached towards a unitary approach to ethnicity and culture in nursing and health care practices, misguided and untested approaches to cultural care will be perpetu-ated in nursing.

Contemporary British writers on cultural care, such as Papadapoulos and Lees (2002), McGee (1992), Narayanasamy and White (2005), to name a few, have adapted and contextualised Leininger's transcultural health care to Brit-ish nursing. These authors develop a discourse that appears to shift away from the factfile and mechanistic features of the culturalist approach. Instead, they appear to offer a holistic approach in which assumptions and stereotypes are challenged within the cultural competence frameworks they have proposed. In its defence, like other meta-narratives, such as the post-colonial and feminism, and like other sociological theorists, contemporary cultural theorists such as Papadapoulos *et al.* and McGee offer a paradigm for cultural dimensions of care with emphasis on the development of cultural competence. Clearly there is a need for research, using the sociological discourses to review the essential-ist approach such as Leininger's nursing and other alternatives. This needs to be done in the context of opposition to multiculturalism (which is increasingly politicised and orchestrated by the media), a rising sense of national identity and xenophobia, fears about Britain being invaded by foreign and inferior cul-tures, and other forms of social division that impact upon people's lives.

Transcultural health care practice and nurse education

Nurse educators can play a prominent role in promoting transcultural care educa-tion. Parfitt (1998, p. 51) suggests that nurse educators can help shape students' attitudes: 'fostering positive attitudes towards patients irrespective of 'race' can introduce programmes to sensitise them to the problems inherent in stereotyp-ing, prejudice and discriminatory practice'. Parfitt calls for a review of the curriculum and the embedding of a programme where ethnicity and cultural concepts are addressed. Likewise, Le Var (1998) offers a review that is systematic with detailed analysis of the problems and offers some remedial solutions. In so doing, Le Var identifies in the health care provisions for transcultural health care: 'language and communication difficulties; lack of information; services not meeting the needs of these clients; misdiagnoses; inappropriate treatments; experiences of racism and racial harassment; lack of equal access to health care services; and diminished service use' (p. 523). Although Le Var's review has far-reaching implications for nurse and health care educators, it could have gone further in exploring the structural and historical location of the problem related to transcultural health care.

However, the general education sector is making some progress in improving racial awareness and promotion of respect and tolerance for people of other ethnicities and cultures, but it will take many generations to reshape attitudes and behaviours. This causes some problems for nurse and other health educators in how realistic it is that the evils of racism and anti-discriminatory practices could be dismantled when their foundations are firmly rooted in attitudes, power and civic structures. Oppressive practices are commonly well disguised and perpetuated to maintain superior status, power relations and positions. However, in spite of these barriers and lifelong processes that perpetuate racism and discrimination, policymakers in education, both general and professional, can work in alliances and partnerships to root out the evils of racism and oppression.

Health carers have voting rights as citizens and therefore hold political influence to demand structural changes to root out the evil of racism, discrimination and oppression. In this respect the Royal College of Nursing (1998) has brought out a clear and authoritative document that suggests the practical ways in which nurses could lobby to bring about changes that improve transcultural health care.

Le Var's paper offers a seven-point plan of action for promoting transcultural health care practices (Table 3.2).

Readers should refer to Le Var (1998, p. 524) for details of the seven-point plan. Le Var argues that in order to put these plans into action, the strategy requires: initiative; enthusiasm; commitment of individuals and groups; strategic planning; organisation and coordination of services; funding; improved education and training of health care professionals; and in-depth knowledge and understanding of, for example, recruitment and research.

Kate Gerrish and Irena Papadopoulos (1999) in their review and analysis of transcultural health care and education, take a more pluralistic approach. They are explicit about anti-racism and assert that transcultural practices based on culturalist approach alone is not satisfactory. They draw attention to the structural factors that have ubiquitous effect on the health experiences of minority ethnic communities These authors stress the need for nurses to understand the complexities of multifactoral issues such as history, politics, social and economic

Table 3.2 Seven-point plan (Le Var, 1998).

1. Development and implementation of local policies and strategies.
2. Removal of language barriers and developing skills in communication with patients and clients and their families.
3. Knowledge development through awareness sessions aimed at eradicating racism.
4. Information on services for users.
5. Development of innovative practices.
6. Involvement of users from ethnic minority groups to develop and improve services.
7. Research to monitor the extent to which the needs of ethnic minority groups for health are being met.

influences on the experiences of minority ethnic communities. They identify a number of other strategies to enable nurses to develop transcultural care competencies. Gerrish and Papadopoulos (1999) suggest that practitioners need to develop both culture-specific and generic cultural competence. Culture-specific competence entails development of knowledge and skills related to a particular ethnic group as well as insights into the beliefs and values that operate within clients' cultures. Such insights are important, as beliefs and values influence clients' perceptions of health, illness and bodily functions. On the other hand, generic cultural competence is about knowledge and skills acquisition that is applicable across ethnic groups.

Innovations in transcultural care practice in nurse education

Gerrish and Papadopoulos (1999) suggest innovative ways of teaching transcultural care practices in nurse education. They stress that the following should feature in the nurse education curriculum: understanding of cultural needs from clients' perspectives and the diversity of interpretations of health and illness that may prevail among different minority ethnic groups; development of communication strategies that are conducive to both carers and users in planning care; an understanding of the influences of socio-economic and political factors in health care delivery systems; and more fundamentally enabling practitioners to be equipped with skills to challenge prejudice, discrimination and inequalities. With regard to practice, these authors advocate the use of expert practitioners from minority ethnic backgrounds to act as role models for learners. This approach can be augmented by students' exposure to examples of innovative transcultural health care practices. These authors also suggest innovative use of information technology to impart knowledge and skills to students on transcultural health care practices. Multimedia materials, video footage, audio recordings, websites, clinical scenarios, simulation exercises are some of the processes of information technology that are indicated as ideal components of nurse educational delivery. Although Gerrish and Papadopoulos offer useful strategies for improving transcultural nursing practice from an educational perspective, there is a need for more specific practical measures for implementing culturally sensitive models of practice.

The ACCESS model for transcultural health care practice

According to Chady (2001), Eisenbruch (2001) and Stanley (2000), the ACCESS Model (Narayanasamy, 2002) offers a framework for transcultural health care practice. The ACCESS Model is represented in Table 3.3. ACCESS as an acronym enables its users to be consciously aware of the various features of this model when applied to the care of minority ethnic patients. Eisenbruch (2001) suggests that the ACCESS model advances 'an alternative to this ethnocentric style of nurse education in cultural competence'.

However, there are radical proposals for cultural competence education. Anderson *et al.* (2003) advocate that cultural safety programmes, as part of transcultural health care education, should use 'post-colonial' and 'post-national feminist' perspectives to reflect on the ways in which race, culture, class, age

Table 3.3 The ACCESS model of transcultural nursing (Narayanasamy, 2002).

Assessment:	Focus on cultural aspects of clients' lifestyle, health beliefs, and health practices.
Communication:	Be aware of variations in verbal and non-verbal responses.
Cultural Negotiation and compromise:	Become more aware of aspects of other people's culture as well as understanding of clients' view and explain their problems.
Establishing respect and rapport:	A therapeutic relation which portrays genuine respect for clients' cultural beliefs and values is required.
Sensitivity:	Deliver diverse culturally sensitive care to culturally diverse groups.
Safety:	Enable clients to derive a sense of cultural safety.

and gender relations operate as subtexts in clinical encounters. They argue that the post- colonial feminist perspective provides critical inquiries with the theoretical lens to examine histories of colonialisation and new forms of colonialism. It also helps us to 'explicate the varied intersecting social relations of people's lives' (p. 211). This model that Anderson *et al*. advocate is particularly relevant in the health care context, in which there has been a legacy of colonialism and imperialism.

In a slightly different vein, writing from a postmodern perspective, Duffy (2001) argues for new, transformative approaches to cultural education. This author is highly critical of current cultural educational programme, embedded in traditional anthropology, as absolute and ignoring the globalisation that impacts the most remote and isolated cultures. Duffy calls for critical reflective analysis in cultural competence education, involving value clarifications: critical examination of one's own culture before focusing on others and their culture. It is speculated that such critical reflective analysis would lead to personal transformations which are characterised by a culturally sensitive approach to the needs of cultural minorities.

Furthermore, Nairn *et al*. (2004) and Foolchand (1995) argue that anti-racist teaching is under-addressed in nurse education. Nairn *et al*. call for explicit measures to embrace anti-racist teaching in nurse education following a critical appraisal of the literature on cultural care education. However, there is a lack of clear direction in these authors' discourse on how this could be achieved in practice. In contrast, Naik (1993) offers a model for anti-racist curriculum in social work education that can be adopted in nurse education. Our view is that there needs to be extensive professional development in anti-racist and cultural competence training for nurse educators before radical proposals are contemplated. Otherwise, the call for anti-racist teaching will continue to be rhetoric ignored within the subtext of racism in the profession.

In a recent study on transcultural health care practice, Narayanasamy (2003) maps out what nurses do to meet the cultural needs of their patients. The findings of this study suggest that although nurses claim to provide cultural care, this is limited to symbolic and concrete aspects of culture, which include responding to religious, dietary, dying and personal care needs. According to this study, there is scope to develop nurses' cultural knowledge and competence through further education. We outline how we are developing nurse education in the light of this study and other research.

Putting transcultural health care education into practice

We provide a brief overview of our approach to transcultural health care education in Nottingham. The ACCESS model (Narayanasamy, 2002) is used as the framework for cultural competence in nurse education programmes at the University of Nottingham. In the recent review of the Diploma in Nursing Course for Pre-Registration Students, we have mapped out the cultural competence contents for the curriculum. We also offer diploma/degree level modules on transcultural health care. Plans are afoot to develop a Diploma/BSc in Transcultural Health Care Studies. In the cultural competence education programmes, students are facilitated to participate in value clarification exercises in developing their self-awareness of personal prejudices, assumptions and stereotypes. They engage in critical reflective thinking and analysis of the effects and impact of racism, ethno-centrism, negative attitudes, cultural imperialism, power relations, discriminatory practices, injustice and disadvantages. They also examine structural factors, such as policies, power, politics and agencies affecting vulnerable and disadvantage groups. The ACCESS model is used to develop cross-cultural communication and cultural negotiations, celebrating diversity and fostering cultural safety. The emphasis of our programme is to enable course participants to make commitments to become agents of change to promote culturally sensitive care through personal transformation. Presently, case studies of participants' implementation of the ACCESS model are progressing. The preliminary findings of these studies are encouraging.

Furthermore, we have set up a Transcultural Health Care Forum for Nurses, other Health Care Professionals and Lecturers. This forum has been proactive in its efforts, enabling members to develop and support good practices related to culturally sensitive care and anti-discriminatory practices. The aims of the forum are to promote:

- Greater awareness related to culture, race and ethnicity in practice and education.
- Good practices related to equal and fair access to appropriate care and treatment for patients.
- Equality of opportunities in all aspects of training, recruitment/retention, promotion and employment of black and minority ethnic staff.

The forum produces newsletters and organises workshops and presentations on transcultural health care practice. Some forum members are leaders in the field of transcultural health care by practice, education and research.

Conclusions

Most of the theoretically driven models of transcultural care are making slow progress in terms of application to practice. However, the emerging literature appears to be promising, with evidence of innovations in cultural care practice and education. The continued pressures on health care practitioners to implement transcultural health care may again perpetuate some of the problems identified earlier, yet transcultural health care practices based on empirically derived knowledge and practice are likely to succeed. However, much of the current understanding on transcultural nursing practice is almost exclusively derived from educational research and literature reviews. A range of perspectives exist with regard to transcultural health care education. This chapter has attempted to highlight the significance of cultural competence education in the context of globalisation, nationalism and postmodernism. Health care professionals have a moral duty to promote cultural competence as a way of eradicating racism and oppressive practices. Each one of the patients is made to be a bright colour in the rich tapestry of life and we need to respect the richness of diversity and differences. We have outlined Nottingham's strategies for cultural competence education in the light of research evidence. However, much practice-based research is needed to accelerate the momentum for changes in practice through research, education and practice, as nursing is primarily about multicultural care in a multi-ethnic society and National Health Service.

References

Acheson, Sir Donald (1998) *The Independent Inquiry into Inequalities in Health.* Stationery Office, London.

Ahmad, W. I. U. (1993) *Race and Health in Contemporary Britain.* Open University Press, Buckingham.

Alleyne, J., Papadopoulos, I. and Tilki, M. (1994) Transcultural care: anti-racism within transcultural nurse education. *British Journal of Nursing,* **3**(12), 635–7.

Anderson, J., Browne, A., Henderson, A., Khan, K. B., Lynam, J., Semeniuk, P. and Smye, V. (2003) 'Rewriting' Cultural safety within the postcolonial and postnational feminist project: toward new epistemologies of healing. *Advances in Nursing Science,* **26**(3), 196–214.

Baxter, C. (2000) Antiracist practice: achieving competency and maintaining professional standards. In: *Lyttle's Mental Health and Disorder* (eds. T. Thompson and P. Mathias), pp. 350–8. Baillière Tindall, Edinburgh.

Bhopal, R. (2001) Racism in medicine. The spectre must be exorcised. *British Medical Journal,* **322**, 1503–4.

Bruni, N. (1988) Critical analysis of transcultural theory. *Australian Journal of Advanced Nursing,* **5**(3), 26–32.

Chady, S. (2001) The NSF for mental health from a transcultural perspective. *British Journal of Nursing*, **10**(15), 984–90.

Cortis, J. D. (2003) Managing society's differences and diversity. *Nursing Standard*, **33**(18), 33–9.

Cortis, J. D. (1993) Transcultural nursing: appropriateness for Britain. *Journal of Advances in Health and Nursing Care*, **12**(4), 67–77.

Culley, L. (2001) Nursing, culture and competence. In: *Ethnicity and Nursing Practice* (eds. L. Culley and S. Dyson), pp. 109–28. Palgrave, Basingstoke.

Department of Health (2000) *The NHS Plan: a Plan for Investment, a Plan for Reform*. Presented to Parliament by the Secretary of State for Health by Command of Her Majesty.

Dobson, S. (1991) *Transcultural Nursing: A Contemporary Imperative*. Scutari, London.

Duffy, M. E. (2001) Journal of Advanced Nursing, **36**(4), 487–95.

Eisenbruch, M. (2001) *National Review of Nursing Education: Multicultural Nursing Education*. Department of Education, Training and Youth Affairs, Commonwealth of Australia.

English National Board (ENB) (1993) *Regulations and Guidelines for the Approval of Institutions and Courses*. English National Board, London.

English National Board (ENB) (1997) *Standards for the Approval of Higher Education Institutions and Programmes*. English National Board, London.

English National Board (ENB) (2000) *Education in Focus, Strengthening Pre-registration Nursing and Midwifery Education*. English National Board, London.

Fernando, S. (1991) *Mental Health, Race and Culture*. Macmillan, London.

Fletcher, M. (1997) Ethnicity: equal health services for all. *Journal of Community Nursing*, **11**(7), 20–4.

Foolchand, M. K. (1995) Promoting racial equality in the nursing curriculum. *Nurse Education Today*, **15**, 101–5.

Foolchand, M. K. (2000) The role of the Department of Health and other key institutions in the provision of equality. *Nurse Education Today*, **20**(6), 443–8.

Friedman, M. K. (1990) Transcultural family nursing: application to Latino and Black families. *Journal of Community Health Nursing*, **8**(1), 33–44.

Gandhi, L. (1998) *Postcolonial Theory. A Critical Introduction*. Columbia University Press, New York.

Gerrish, K. and Papadopoulos, I. (1999) Transcultural competence: the challenge for nurse education. *British Journal of Nursing*, **8**(21), 1453–7.

Gerrish, K., Husband, C. and Mackenzie, J. (1996) *Nursing for a Multi-Ethnic Society*. Open University Press, Buckingham.

Gilroy, P. (2000) *Against Race: Imaging Political Culture Beyond the Color Line*. The Belknap Press of Harvard University Press, Cambridge.

Gunaratnam, Y. (1997) Culture is not enough: a critique of multiculturalism in palliative care. In: *Death, Gender and Ethnicity* (eds. D. Field, J. Hockey and N. Small), pp. 166–86. Routledge, London.

Guibernau, M. and Goldblatt, D. (2000) Identity and nation. In: *Questioning Identity: Gender, Class, Nation* (ed. K. Woodward). Routledge/Open University, London.

Henley, A. and Schott, J. (1999) *Culture, Religion and Patient Care in a Multi-Ethnic Society*. Age Concern, London.

Herberg, P. (1989) Theoretical foundations of transcultural nursing. In: *Transcultural Concepts in Nursing Care* (J. S. Boyle and M. M. Andrews), pp. 3–53. Scott, Foresman/Little, Brown College Division, Illinois.

Hofstede, G. (1991) *Cultures and Organisation – the Software of the Mind*. McGraw-Hill, London.

Holland, K. and Hogg, C. (2001) *Cultural Awareness in Nursing and Health Care: An Introductory Text*. Arnold, London.

Kavanagh, K. (1995) Transcultural perspectives in mental health. In: *Transcultural Concepts in Nursing Care*, 2nd edn (eds. M. M. Anderson and J. S. Boyle), pp. 253–85. J. P. Lippincott Co., Philadelphia.

Kerslake, M. (1988) Across cultures. *New Zealand Journal*, January, 20–22.

Leininger, M. (1997a) Transcultural nursing research to nursing education and practice: 40 years. *Image Journal of Nursing Scholarship*, **29**(4), 341–7.

Leininger, M. (1997b) *Transcultural Nursing: Concepts, Theories and Practice*. John Wiley, Chichester.

Leininger, M. (2001) A mini journey into transcultural nursing with its founder. *Nebraska Nurse*, **34**(2), 16–17.

Le Var, R. M. H. (1998) Improving educational preparation for transcultural health care. *Nurse Education Today*, **18**, 519–33.

Littlewood, R. and Lipsedge, M. (1981) *Aliens and Alienists: Ethnic Minorities and Psychiatry*. Penguin, London.

Macdonald, J. (1987) Preparing to work in a multicultural society (in Canada). *Canadian Nurse/Informière Canadienne*, **83**, 31–2.

Macpherson, Sir William (1999) *The Stephen Lawrence Inquiry*. Stationery Office, London.

McGee, P. (1992) *Issues in Transcultural Nursing: a Guide for Teachers of Nursing and Health*. Chapman & Hall, London.

Modood, T. (1992) *Not Easy Being British: Colour, Culture and Citizenship*. Runnymede Trust and Trentham Books, London.

Naik, D. (1993) Towards an anti-racist curriculum in social work training. In: *Health, Welfare and Practice* (eds. J. Walmsley, J. Reynolds, P. Shakespeare and R. Woolfe). Open University, Milton Keynes.

Nairn, S., Hardy, C., Parumal, L. and Williams, G. (2004) Multicultural or anti-racist teaching in nurse education: a critical appraisal. *Nurse Education Today*, **24**, 188–95.

Narayanasamy, A. (1998) *Religious, Spiritual and Cultural Resource Package.* University of Nottingham/Queen's Medical Centre, Nottingham.

Narayanasamy, A. (1999a) Transcultural mental health nursing 1: benefits and limitations. *British Journal of Nursing*, **8**(11), 664–8.

Narayanasamy, A. (1999b) Transcultural mental health nursing 2: race, ethnicity and culture. *British Journal of Nursing*, **8**(12), 741–4.

Narayanasamy, A. (2000) Cultural impact of Islam on the future directions of nurse education. *Nurse Education Today*, **20**, 57–64.

Narayanasamy, A. (2002) The ACCESS model: a transcultural nursing practice framework. *British Journal of Nursing*, **11**(9), 643–50.

Narayanasamy, A. (2003) Transcultural nursing: how do nurses respond to cultural needs? *British Journal of Nursing*, **12**(2), 36–45.

Narayanasamy, A. and White, E. (2005) A review of transcultural nursing. *Nurse Education Today*, **25**, 102–11.

National Health Service Executive (NHSE) (1999) *Tackling Racial Harassment in the NHS. A Plan for Action.* Department of Health, London.

Papadopoulos, I., Tilki, M. and Taylor, G. (1998) *Transcultural Care: A Guide for Health Care Professionals.* Quay, Wiltshire.

Papadopoulos, I. and Lees, I. (2002) Developing culturally competent research. *Journal of Advanced Nursing*, **37**(3), 258–63.

Parfitt, B. (1998) *Working Across Culture: A Study of Expatriate Nurses Working in Developing Countries in Primary Health Care.* Ashage, Aldershot.

Peberdy, A. (1997) Communicating across cultural boundaries. In: *Debates and Dilemmas in Promoting Health: A Reader* (eds. M. Siddle, L. Jones, J. Katz and A. Peberdy), pp. 99–107. Open University, Buckinghamshire.

Polachek, N. R. (1998) Cultural safety: a new concept in nursing people of different ethnicities. *Journal of Advanced Nursing*, **27**(3), 452–7.

The Quality Assurance Agency for Higher Education (2001) *Benchmark Statement: Health Care Programmes.* London.

Qureshi, B. (1989) *Transcultural Medicine.* Kluwer Academic, Dordrecht.

Rassool, G. H. (1995) The health status and health care of ethno-cultural minorities in the United Kingdom: an agenda for action. *Journal of Nursing*, **21**, 199–201.

Rack, P. (1990) Psychological/psychiatric disorders. In: *Health Care for Asians* (eds. B. R. McAvoy and L. J. Donaldson), pp. 290–303. Routledge, London.

Rothenburger, R. (1990) Transcultural nursing: overcoming obstacles to effective communication. *AORN Journal*, **51**(5), 1349–52.

Royal College of Nursing (RCN) (1998) *The Nursing Care of Older People From Black and Minority Ethnic Communities*. Royal College of Nursing, London.

Sawley, L. (2001) Perceptions of racism in the health service. *Nursing Standard*, **15**(19), 33–5.

Serrant Green, L. (2001) Transcultural nursing education: a view from within. *Nurse Education Today*, **21**(8), 670–8.

Stanley, S. (2000) Commentary: the cultural impact of Islam on the future direction of nurse education. *Nurse Education Today*, **20**(1), 69.

Stokes, G. (1991) A transcultural nurse is about. *Senior Nurse*, **11**(1), 40–2.

Thomas, V. and Dines, V. (1994) The health care needs of ethnic minorities groups: are nurses and individuals playing their part? *Journal of Advanced Nursing*, **20**, 802–8.

United Kingdom Central Council for Nursing, Midwifery and Health Visiting (UKCC) (1999) *Fitness for Practice*. The UKCC Commission for Nursing and Midwifery Education. Chair: Sir Leonard Peach. UKCC, London.

Wilkins, H. (1993) Transcultural nursing: a selective review of the literature, 1985–1991. *Journal of Advanced Nursing*, **18**, 602–16.

Wright, J. (1991) Counselling at the cultural interface: is getting back to roots enough? *Journal of Advanced Nursing*, **16**, 92–100.

CHAPTER 4

Spiritual coping mechanisms in chronically ill patients

Summary

Addressing spiritual needs is acknowledged as an essential component of holistic nursing care. Findings are emerging that suggest that chronic illness demands significant changes in patients' lifestyles. In such circumstances it is claimed that spiritual care can be therapeutic to patients (Cohen *et al.*, 2000; Sherwood, 2000). This study was carried out in order to understand further the spiritual coping mechanisms of patients suffering from chronic illness. A qualitative methodology based on descriptive phenomenology was used to capture participants' lived experience. The main themes emerging from this study suggest that chronic illness leads participants to use the following spiritual coping mechanisms: faith, prayer and related sources of support. Patients coping with chronic illness were engaged in both personal and private struggles. Patients may benefit from nursing interventions that are sensitive, supportive and responsive to their spiritual needs.

Key points

- Spirituality is an essential component of holistic nursing care.
- Qualitative inquiry illuminates the phenomenon of spiritual coping mechanisms.
- Spirituality can be vital as a coping mechanism for chronically ill patients.
- Beliefs and faith, prayer and the search for meaning and purpose, privacy with regard to spiritual practices and sources of support are important spiritual coping mechanisms.
- Nursing interventions should be sensitive, supportive, and responsive to patients' spiritual needs.

Introduction

Addressing spiritual needs is acknowledged as an essential component of holistic nursing care. In the literature, holistic care is described as care of the body, mind and spirit (Narayanasamy, 1999). One study suggests that the diagnosis of chronic illness in patients is a critical juncture in life which demands significant changes in lifestyle (Aldridge, 1987). In such circumstances it is claimed that spiritual care can be therapeutic to patients (Cohen *et al.*, 2000; Sherwood, 2000). Although the significance of spirituality in patients' lives as they face illness is acknowledged in the emerging health care literature, there is a paucity of literature and research with regard to the lived experience of spiritual coping mechanisms in chronically ill patients in the UK. The purpose of this study was to open this area of research by exploring the lived experience of spiritual coping mechanisms in a community of chronically ill patients.

This chapter provides a literature review on spirituality and spiritual needs in chronic illness. It identifies the gap in the literature on the lived experience of spiritual coping mechanisms in chronically ill clients. Following a discussion on methodological issues and analysis, the lived experience of spiritual coping mechanisms in chronic illness is illuminated. The insights derived from this study may help nurses to be sensitive and responsive to the spiritual needs of chronically ill patients.

Literature review

Spirituality and nursing

Health-related literature has begun to highlight spirituality and its importance in health and illness. Spirituality is described as a dimension of being human which gives individuals a sense of being, with qualities that include innateness (Chandler *et al.*, 1992), a capacity for inner knowing, and a source of strength (Burkhardt, 1994), subjective experience of the sacred (Vaughan, 1995), self-transcendence towards a capacity for greater love and knowledge (Chandler *et al.*, 1992), a unity or wholeness permeating all of one's life (Burkhardt, 1994), and provision of meaning of one's existence that lies at the core of one's being. Further, in the developing discourse on spirituality, scholars appear to converge on two points. First, humans are seen as spiritual beings, and second, there is a connection between spirituality and healing. With regard to humans as spiritual beings, Fry (1997) states 'spirituality is a profound and central aspect of the existence of many people', leading to the claim that spirituality and nursing are intertwined in the lived experience of people in terms of nurse–patient interactions (Fry, 1997). With regard to spirituality and healing, there is a consensus in the literature about the influence of spirituality on the power of recovery and the ability to cope with and adjust to the varying and demanding states of health and illness (Bradshaw, 1994; Fry, 1997; Ross, 1997; McSherry, 2000; Narayanasamy, 2001).

Definition of spirituality

The literature on nursing places an emphasis on spirituality. From a holistic perspective, such literature describes spirituality or spiritual life in the terms listed in Table 4.1.

Although spirituality is the essence of our being, its depth and intensity vary between individuals. Sherwood (2000) points out the ambiguity between the terms 'spirituality' and 'religion', and attributes this ambiguity to blurring of the concepts. The distinctiveness of these concepts is acknowledged in the literature; however, Cohen *et al.* (2000) suggest that the religious dimension may be one component of spirituality. Illness and other crises compel some individuals to turn to religion and seek comfort in its tenets and traditions. For some it seems that religion can be a source of support in terms of 'hope and guidance in enabling individuals to examine their spirituality, define their purpose in life, and connect with a community' (Cohen *et al.*, 2000).

Spiritual needs

There are variations in the definitions of spiritual needs owing to the influence of the belief systems and values of the various authors (MacKinlay, 2001; Narayanasamy, 2001). The theoretical perspectives of the present study are derived from contemporary sources such as Reed (1992), Bradshaw (1994), Narayanasamy (1999), Cohen *et al.* (2000) and Sherwood (2000). Such literature espouses that, in the main, spiritual needs are characterised by normal expressions of a person's inner being that motivates the search for meaning in all experiences and a dynamic relationship with others, self, and whatever the person values. Spiritual needs may be attained through faith, hope, love, trust, meaning and purpose, relationships, forgiveness, creativity, and experiences. These qualities are important for our holistic wellbeing in terms of meaningful existence. Some people achieve these via religious beliefs and practices (Sherwood, 2000).

Table 4.1 Descriptions of spirituality.

- The essence or life principle of person (Clark *et al.*, 1991)
- A sacred journey (Mische, 1982)
- The experience of the radical truth of things (Legere, 1984) and ultimate values (Cawley, 1997)
- Giving meaning and purpose in life (Legere, 1984; Clark *et al.*, 1991; Fitchett, 1995; Sherwood, 2000)
- Relating to unconditional love (Ellison, 1983; Clark *et al.*, 1991; Ross, 1997)
- Connectedness within oneself (Reed, 1992) and others (Sherwood, 2000)
- A life relationship or a sense of connection with mystery, a Higher Power, God or Universe (Granstrom, 1985; Reed, 1992)
- A belief that relates a person to the world (Soeken and Carson, 1987)
- A quality that invokes a need to transcend the self in such a way that empowers, not devalues, the individual (Sherwood, 2000)
- Inner dimension of being human attuned to the most valuable aspect of life that motivates and guides one's significant choices (Emblen, 1992)
- Being rooted in an awareness which is part of the biological makeup of the human species (Narayanasamy, 1999)
- Referring to meaning and unity, and a Transcendent, usually referred to as God in the West (Aldridge, 2000)
- That which gives meaning, purpose, hope and value to people's lives. This is part of a wide concept which may include, but is not defined by, religious faith and culture (Swinton, 2002).

Chronic illness and spirituality

Knowledge related to chronic illness and nursing has emerged (Werner-Boland, 1980; Lewis, 1985), but the literature on spirituality and chronic illness is rather scarce. Miller (1983) refers to chronic illness as 'an altered health state that will not be cured by a surgical procedure or a short course of medical therapy'. The person with chronic illness may experience a range of impaired functioning involving the body, mind and spirit, and the perpetual illness-related demands on self. Fieldman (1974) considers chronic illness as a new altered 'state of being' in that it is impossible for clients to view themselves and life as before. The illness permeates the person's whole being until it does not leave any part of life untouched, taking over the person's body, mind and spirit, relationships, roles and lifestyle. Narayanasamy (1996) and Kitson (1985) provide some guidance to nurses on the spiritual care of chronically ill patients. This literature emphasises that nurses can adopt roles as comforters, counsellors and advocates in enabling chronically ill patients to meet their spiritual needs. Although this approach may be useful, there is scope to develop this further in the light of empirical evidence related to practice.

Researchers investigating spirituality and chronic illness have found spirituality to be a powerful resource for coping with health-related problems. Yates *et al.* (1981) found that religion acted as an important source of support for many patients. Baldree *et al.* (1982) assessed the methods of coping used by 35 haemodialysis patients and found that hope, prayer and trust in God were prominent coping mechanisms. In another study, Miller (1983) found that arthritis patients reported a significantly higher level of religious wellbeing in relation to God. Likewise, Johnson and Spilka (1991) found that prayer and faith were extremely important resources for the majority of cancer patients who participated in their study.

Fernsler *et al.* (1999) found that people with colorectal cancer who reported higher levels of spiritual wellbeing had significantly lower demands of illness in relation to physical and monitoring symptoms and treatment issues. In the light of their findings, these researchers suggest that a greater degree of spiritual wellbeing may help to mitigate the demands of illness as a consequence of colorectal cancer.

In a spirituality and bone marrow transplantation study, Cohen *et al.* (2000) found that through personal stories, participants sought opportunities for reflections, including adjustment to loss and resolutions. Spirituality and spiritual support from nurses appeared to have been instrumental to the adjustment and resolutions achieved by patients.

Many of the above research findings have emerged from North American studies and there is a problem in applying the significance of the above findings to UK health care practice, as the context and nature of suffering in chronic illness may be different (as may the experience of lived spirituality). Furthermore, many of these studies involve quantitative methods investigating correlations between spiritual factors and outcomes, leading to adjustment to illness. Such measures may fail to capture the lived experiences of patients suffering from chronic illness. Accounts of spiritual coping mechanisms from a community of sufferers in the UK may provide much contextual evidence to inform practice.

Aim of the study

The aim of this study was to describe the lived experience of spiritual coping mechanisms in participants who were chronically ill.

Methods

The study used descriptive phenomenology (Husserl, 1989) and involved unstructured interviews with 15 chronically ill patients. Descriptive phenomenology as a qualitative approach is suited to find out about human lived experiences of their health, illness and nursing (Ashworth, 1997a,b; Derbyshire, 1997). In respect to the qualitative approach, Ashworth (1997a) advances that it is the responsibility of the researcher to reveal clearly the reality of life as experienced by participants. The sample was purposive, based on potential participants' abilities to identify and discuss openly their experiences of spiritual coping while facing chronic illness. Adult patients having had a chronic illness for six months were included in the study. For the purpose of this study chronic illness is defined as 'an altered health state that will not be cured by a surgical procedure or a short course of medical therapy' (Miller, 1983). Only those patients who were psychologically and physically able were included in this study. These selection criteria ensured that the patients were in a stable physical and mental state to make informed decisions about participating in the research and being interviewed. A further consideration was that as all participants had experienced the illness for six months or longer, they would be able to provide detailed accounts of their lived experience of spiritual coping mechanisms.

Several patients were approached and 15 of them (10 men and five women) agreed to participate. Their ages ranged from 23–80 years. With regard to patients' religious status, nine claimed to be Christians and two identified themselves as Hindus; the remaining four claimed to have no specific religious affiliation. Their medical diagnosis included leukaemia, melia fibrosis, bowel cancer, chronic liver disease, Crohn's disease, lung cancer, ulcerative colitis and melanoma. The participants were hospitalised for a variety of treatments and procedures, including chemotherapy and symptom control.

Following permission from the ethical committee of the institution, participants were approached by the researcher, who made appointments with them for interview at a time and place convenient to them. Participants were asked to talk about their experiences related to their illness, and how they coped from the point of diagnosis to present medical treatment and care. All responses were tape-recorded and participants were encouraged to describe fully their experiences, feelings and thoughts. Clarification related to responses was sought at appropriate times during the course of the interview, but caution was exercised to avoid suggestive and leading questions. The interviews lasted between 45 and 90 minutes.

Data analysis

The phenomenological method of analysis adapted from Colaizzi (1983) and Haase (1987) was used (Table 4.2). The data analysis involved a process in which the investigator developed a sense of feeling for and familiarity with participants' accounts of their experience by listening to the whole tape-recordings several times and transcribing them verbatim. Participants described their coping mechanism from the time of their diagnosis to the present. Examples included the point at which they were informed of their diagnosis for the first time (6–12 months ago), the feelings this news evoked in them and the steps they had to take to cope, adjusting to the news and the impact of the illness and so on. Each transcript was read and re-read to develop an understanding of the emerging themes and meaning.

As suggested by Ashworth (1997b), the data gathering was treated as 'a process of discovery, concentrating in the first instance on each individual as a separate case, a possibly unique world'. At the initial stage of the analysis due care was taken to avoid making assumptions about the emerging themes, as each case is unique and assumptions that the meanings of the same situation are similar for different people should not be made.

As the analysis progressed, recurrent themes related to participants' spiritual coping mechanisms emerged (see Table 4.3 for examples). The themes were integrated into a description of participants' experience. The emphasis here was

Table 4.2 Data analysis: Colaizzi's eight-step analytical process.

1. Acquisition of a sense of each protocol's meaning through listening to and transcribing the tapes
2. Extracting of significant statements
3. Formulation of significant statements into a more general statement
4. Formulation of a statement of meaning and validation of that meaning by judges
5. Organisation of formulated meanings into themes, theme clusters, and theme categories
6. Integration of themes into an exhaustive description of phenomena of interest
7. Formulation of the statement of the essential structure
8. Validation of the essential structure by study participants

Table 4.3 Examples of categories, theme clusters and themes.

Category	Theme cluster	Themes
Reaching out to God in the belief and faith that help will be forthcoming	A plea for divine power to intervene An awareness of a presence	Faith in God, calling for help from God, a private call for help from someone out there, being close to God, the threat of death forced... seek help... Feeling the presence of someone than self, a comforting presence, being looked after...
Feeling connected to God through prayer	Making a plea to God	Making plea to God, asking for God's favour, asking God to help me and my family, calling to rescue me...
	Submitting everything to God	Submitting to God's will, committing everything to God, leaving everything to God, fasting and praying...
	Dialogue with God	Having a dialogue with God, a relationship and communication with God, ... someone out there, arguing and telling Him off... keeping Him informed, talking to Him...
	Feeling uplifted and hopeful	Feeling comforted, relief, confidence, deriving special strength, feeling helped, a sense of feeling good and feeling a sense of being lifted...
Meaning and purpose	Reflections and contemplation	Meaning of life and purpose, directions, thinking about nature, questions about life and impact of illness, existence...
Strategy of privacy	Private and personal nature of experience	Fear of being ridiculed, privacy, feelings, concealment, sense of loneliness, conflicts, unresolved issues...
Connectedness with others	Sources of support	Family relationships, friendship, fellowship, spiritual resources, visits, contacts, religious agents...

to represent participants' experience of chronic illness and coping mechanisms in terms of their beliefs.

Findings: the experience of spiritual coping mechanisms

According to the participants, chronic illness is an experience in which they resorted to coping mechanisms, some of which appear to be spiritual in nature. These are described below.

Reaching out to God in the belief and faith that help will be forthcoming

As participants lived their experience of coping spiritually with their chronic illness, they reached out to God in the belief and faith that help would be forthcoming to rescue them from the illness. A patient shared his experience:

> When they told me that I have cancer the news devastated me. I started to think about myself, my family and the future. I thought to myself what have I done to deserve this... it was terrible, I felt numb, confused, bewildered.... Obviously, you feel terrible, who wouldn't in this situation...? Then I started to think of the power above us.... So I called for a Divine Power, in a way calling God to come and rescue me from this mess, if you like... you can say it is a sort of a belief in God to bail me out, really.

For some chronically ill patients, the news of their diagnosis might be the first time they have experienced a spiritual need:

> ... that was the first time I started to think if there is a God, and I began to plead to Him to help me during this crisis... you may think I am silly but that is my way of dealing with this problem. When you are well you never think about things like this, do you?

Participants also reflected that their faith gave them further strength to cope with the crisis. A patient reflected:

> ... my belief that God is in ultimate control and can help me find relief in my suffering is a great source of strength and comfort.

Another patient shared a similar experience:

> I suppose my faith will remain stronger. I am lucky that God is with me, he helps me through. I have heard of others being not so lucky as they had to face extreme suffering

The connection with God is so intense that some participants talked about an awareness of a presence they felt. A patient disclosed:

> People would think that I am making it up, they would think that I am going funny but I felt that someone was present... it was comforting that I am being looked after...

Feeling connected to God through prayer

Some participants reflected that they felt connected to God through prayer. These participants' experience is that they wanted to be closer to God, to feel his presence, and felt that they could in part bring that about by praying. Prayer was used as a private and personal resource in communicating with God in order to cope with their chronic illnesses:

> I frequently make a plea to God in my prayer to ask Him to come and help me, help me to get through the night... night time is a real problem for me as things keep coming back to my mind. I then turn to my prayers, I say to Him, please, please help me sleep through the night.

The suffering as a result of chronic illness led some patients to connect to God through prayer as a dialogue to cope with crisis:

> ... when I pray I have a dialogue with God... I tell Him everything that is happening to me. It's like talking to a friend who listens... I can unload my problems. This dreadful illness, the pain... sometimes, I tell Him off for letting me down... prayer helps me, knowing that there is someone out there who listens.

Another patient shared his experience that he submitted everything to God as a way of connecting:

> In my prayers, I submit everything to God, He knows that I'm suffering and He will help me to get through the crisis. He has responded to me, answered my prayers, although I don't feel this at times... I have a deep faith, my prayers will help me, I submit the lot to Him.

Some participants implied that the connection with God through prayer had helped them to feel uplifted and hopeful:

> I felt uplifted and hopeful as I know the Lord has listened to me. I feel reassured that there is someone there to help me...

Another patient shared a similar experience:

> I feel that I'm supported by God, I know there is a God who supports me, a God I haven't seen, but I'm supported... I suppose it's my belief in God

The search for meaning and purpose

Participants' descriptions of their experience revealed episodes characterising reflections and contemplations about the meaning and purpose of life:

> ... my faith, work, my family and friends... nature provides meaning and purpose for me, I think. I find that things to do with nature [are] intensely inspiring and these give me a sense of meaning.... Sometimes, I feel that all these things give meaning for my very existence... my illness challenges all these... the adaptation I've had to make. I like walking but now I will only go out on a good day... Yes, when I feel up to it...

A strategy of privacy

Participants' reflections about their experience of coping extended to disclosures about personal fears and the privacy of their experiences. Participants adopted a strategy of keeping their spiritual coping mechanism as a private and personal affair. Spiritual experiences and practices such as awareness of a 'presence' or attempts to connect with God through prayers were largely kept private. Privacy extends further than concealment from a visiting researcher and may even include close family members:

> ... I keep this private, I pray quietly as I feel my beliefs are very private... there is no point in letting others know about this... some people would turn around and say what's the matter with him, he has gone funny or gone mental as well.

Connectedness with others

In the absence of apparent forms of spiritual care, participants expressed a need to be connected with others who are seen as sources of spiritual support for them: their family, friends, church ministers and religious fellowships:

> My family is a good source of support... when I was taken ill, apart from my wife and children, my brothers and sisters, when they heard of my illness, they travelled to be around us... they prayed, prayed intensely for my recovery.

On occasions when therapeutic spiritual support was expected but not forth-coming, for some participants the spiritual need became a lonely struggle. A patient observed:

... the ward did not offer much in the way of my spiritual need... how-ever, they did respect me as an individual, treated me with respect and dignity, but they did not ask if I wanted a priest or not. I wasn't in a position to ask for one either, but would have liked to be informed if there is one... as I said before, somehow, I managed prayers on my own.

However, it is worth noting that not all patients welcomed spiritual care interventions. One participant disclosed that a member of the chaplaincy staff approached her uninvited while she was in hospital. She felt distressed about this intrusion and the last thing she wanted was the presence of a religious person. This patient recounted:

I was distressed to find a person from the chaplaincy wanting to talk to me about my religion. He just appeared without asking me

The opportunity to be connected with others means that support networks, such as family relationships, friendship, and church/religious affiliations, are important coping mechanisms during chronic illness.

Discussion

The findings of this study illuminate some of the spiritual coping mechanisms of patients with chronic illness. It appears that, as part of their inner experience, patients reached out to God in the belief and faith that help would be forth-coming to rescue them from the illness. In this respect, faith, that is, belief in a Divine figure, appears to be an integral part of spiritual coping mechanisms during the course of chronic illness.

Aden (1974), Fowler (1974) and Westerhoff (1976) advanced the notion that faith is a universal phenomenon. Miller (1983), Benson and Stark (1996) and Sherwood (2000) identify the power of faith and its influences on healing. Therefore the lived experience of participants in this study is revealing in that a belief in the power of the divinity is possibly a source of strength that gives courage and hope as they face demands of chronic illness. The power of hope as an effective coping mechanism during suffering and uncertainty is well illus-trated in the literature (Herth and Cutcliffe, 2002).

Emerging empirical evidence suggests that hope serves to nourish people in many ways in difficult times. In the present study, the participants' experience of hope as divine intervention to rescue could be seen as normal and functional to existence (Kubler-Ross, 1975).

Another revealing aspect of this study is that some participants' inner experience was so intense that they felt a presence. Empirical studies of spiritual experience suggest that almost half of the British adult population believe that they have been spiritually aware, at least from time to time (Hay, 1987). Drawing from the work of Otto (1950), Hardy (1979) and James (1982), Hay characterises this awareness as feeling a presence; usually this experience is defined in the Western world as an awareness of God. It would seem premature to speculate about this phenomenon in the absence of further empirical evidence of this nature in the clinical context. However, it is significant that those participants who have had experiences of this nature described that they felt comforted, and that they were being looked after.

A further revealing aspect of this study is that some participants felt that they connected to God through prayer. Prayer was used as a private and personal resource in communicating with God in order to cope with their chronic illnesses. Scholars have written extensively about the therapeutic value of prayer (Sodestrom and Martinson, 1987; Bearon and Koenig, 1990; Gustafson, 1992; Benson and Stark, 1996; Aldridge, 2000). Gustafson (1992) illustrates the petitionary and supplication nature of prayers, and more recently Aldridge (2000) highlighted the therapeutic values of meditative, intercessory and liturgical prayers. In the present study participants reflected that they had used prayers of transaction ('when I pray I have a dialogue with God'), petition ('make a plea to God in my prayer') and submission ('in my prayers, I submit everything to God'). According to Aldridge (2000), the search for evidence in support of prayer may prove to be difficult. However, in the present study evidence shows that participants felt uplifted and hopeful, and derived special strength when they prayed.

Although the findings of this study are indicative rather than conclusive, there is scope for further research to explore whether various forms of prayers as a spiritual activity may complement health care and treatment as a source of comfort and support. The healing effects of intercessory prayers (prayer for others), are well documented (Byrd, 1988; Dossey, 1999; Swinton, 2000). However, Swinton (2000) points out that the research on the healing power of prayer is inconclusive and he calls for extensive empirical investigations in this area of spirituality.

Apart from the need for reaching out to God to be rescued and connection with God through prayer, spiritual pursuits in the sense of meaning and purpose appear to be significant in the lives of chronically ill patients. Such reappraisal may be focused on issues of purpose for being and meaning in illness and suffering (Fitchett, 1995; Sherwood, 2000). The implications of this in health or ill health are that personal meaning systems are challenged and intensify further the search to make sense of life in both believers and non-believers. Dickinson (1975) suggests that those positive meanings in life are commonly found in anyone, in spite of the severity of their illness. This search for meaning and purpose can provide a sense of peace, tranquillity and resolution for some people.

Furthermore, the findings illuminate that participants' experience of coping extended to disclosures about personal fears and the need for privacy. For fear of ridicule, participants' concealment about their inner spiritual experiences not only extended to carers, but may also even include close family members. This aspect of the findings reveals that spirituality has its heart in personal and private experience. Concealment about spiritual beliefs and practices became necessary to prevent ridicule about them. Simsen (1986) makes this point about patients' reluctance to disclose their religious concerns, in her study of patients' spiritual care in a hospital:

> ... patients learn that it's fine to talk about bedpans and bowels, but their fears and religious concern – are far less acceptable conversation topics.

Within the general British population, Hay (1987) found in his study of religious experience that people tend to admit shyly to having had religious experience and fear that they are in a minority, and will be thought by most people as stupid or mentally unbalanced. So it is not surprising that patients similarly tend to keep this very private.

However, an observation of this research is that during interviews, although initially reticent, participants were willing to discuss their spiritual beliefs and practices when prompted and encouraged. This suggests that although they fear that there is a taboo, once they discover that there are supportive listeners when they talk of spirituality, patients are usually articulate and keen to talk.

Another significant aspect of participant experience is that when anticipated spiritual support was not forthcoming, the spiritual need became a lonely struggle. In such circumstances, a sense of connectedness with others appears to be an important coping mechanism. Participants' families, friends, church ministers, and religious fellowships were perceived as important sources of support and connectedness. The literature identifies that sources of support provide the opportunities for being connected with others (Narayanasamy, 2000).

An important part of the individuals' spirituality is the sense of connectedness with God and others. Estrangement from them may lead to spiritual distress. Sherwood (2000) suggests that an attitude of hope and talking with others helps sufferers to deal with their emotions as they connect with others who understand them. This in turn may lead to healing, i.e. restoration of the harmonious balance between the body, mind, and spirit (Aldridge, 2000; Swinton, 2002). Further evidence about the phenomenon of connectedness with others as a spiritual coping mechanism is lacking in the literature. However, the revelation in the present study about connectedness with others is possibly indicative of a spiritual coping mechanism. Further research on the phenomenon of connectedness with others as a spiritual coping mechanism is needed before conclusions are drawn.

Conclusion

This chapter illuminates that for the clients in this study chronic illness may become a 'spiritual encounter' as well as a physical and emotional experience. Of significance is the fact that this study reveals that the lived experience of connectedness with God and others, and the search for meaning and purpose, appear to be important spiritual coping mechanisms during chronic illness. The experience of chronic illness may evoke a need in some patients to reach out to God in the belief and faith that help will be forthcoming to rescue them from the illness. Sometimes this intense need leads to the experience of a felt Divine presence which appears to be spiritual resource that offers reassuring prospects that people would be helped through the crisis brought on by the illness. The patients' needs to be connected with God were established through prayers of petition, transaction and submission as spiritual coping mechanisms. Furthermore, a sense of hope, strength, and security may derive from prayer.

The trajectory of chronic illness evokes a need for spiritual pursuits in terms of the search for meaning and purpose. This search is characterised by contemplation about the meaning of life, with positive consequences such as a sense of peace and tranquillity. Aspects of coping strategies, such as communicating with a Divine figure and feeling a Divine presence, are kept as private encounters with efforts to conceal them from others. This concealment is necessary for fear of being ridiculed if found out. When overt therapeutic support related to their spiritual need is not available, patients continue to reflect a desire to be connected with other sources of support such as networks of families and friends. However, a point of consideration is that not all participants welcome spiritual resources of a religious nature. This study offers only a partial picture with regard to the spiritual coping mechanisms in that a majority of patients who participated in the study were adherents of religious faiths. Much research is needed in a variety of clinical settings to map out the specific nature of spiritual coping mechanisms in both believers and non-believers. There is scope for further studies using both qualitative and quantitative methods to provide greater insights into spiritual coping mechanisms.

Acknowledgements

This study is the larger part of a project on spiritual care research sponsored by Trinity Care, part of the Southern Cross Healthcare Group. My thanks are extended to all participants in the study and external and internal reviewers for their valuable comments.

References

Aden, L. (1974) Faith and the development cycle. *Pastoral Psychology*, **28**(2), 215–30.

Aldridge, D. (1987) Families, cancer and dying. *Family Practice*, **4**(3), 212–18.

Aldridge, D. (2000) *Spirituality, Healing and Medicine*. Jessica Kingsley, London.

Ashworth, P. (1997a) The variety of qualitative research. Part one: Introduction to the problem. *Nurse Education Today*, **17**, 215–18.

Ashworth, P. (1997b) The variety of qualitative research. Part two: Non-positivist approaches. *Nurse Education Today*, **17**, 219–24.

Baldree, K. S., Murphy, S. P. and Powers, M. J. (1982) Stress identification and coping patterns in patients on hemodialysis. *Nursing Research*, **31**, 107–10.

Bearon, L. and Koenig, H. (1990) Religious cognitions and use of prayer in health and illness. *Gerontologist*, **30**, 249–53.

Benson, H. and Stark, M. (1996) *Timeless Healing: The Power of Biology of Belief*. Simon & Schuster, London.

Bradshaw, A. (1994) *Lighting the Lamp: The Spiritual Dimension of Nursing Care*. Scutari Press, London.

Burkhardt, M. A. (1994) Becoming and connecting: elements of spirituality for women. *Holist Nursing Practice*, **8**(4), 12–21.

Byrd, R. C. (1988) Positive therapeutic effects of intercessory prayer in a coronary care unit population. *Southern Medical Journal*, **81**(7), 826–9.

Cawley, N. (1997) Towards defining spirituality: an exploration of the concept of spirituality. *International Journal of Palliative Nursing*, **3**(1), 31–6.

Chandler, C. K., Holden, J. M. and Kolander, C. A. (1992) Counselling for spiritual wellness: theory and practice. *Journal of Counselling and Development*, **171**, 169–75.

Clark, C. C., Cross, J. R., Deane, D. M. and Lowery, L. W. (1991) Spirituality: integral to quality care. *Holistic Nursing Practice*, **5**(3), 67–76.

Cohen, Z., Headley, J. and Sherwood, G. W. (2000) Spirituality and bone marrow transplantation: when faith is stronger than fear. *International Journal for Human Caring*, **4**(2), 40–6.

Colaizzi, P. F. (1983) Psychological research as the phenomenologist views it. In: *Existentialist Alternatives for Psychology* (eds. R. S. Valle and M. Kind). Oxford University Press, New York.

Derbyshire, P. (1997) Qualitative research: is it becoming a new orthodoxy? *Nursing Inquiry*, **4**(1), 1–2.

Dickinson, C. (1975) The search for meaning. *American Journal of Nursing*, **75**(10), 1789–93.

Dossey, L. (1999) God in the laboratory: a look at science, prayer, and healing. *The Oates Journal*, Vol. 2. Wayne. E Oates Institute, Kentucky. http://www.oates.org/journal/mbr/vol-02-99/articles/dossey-01.htm

Ellison, C. W. (1983) Spiritual wellbeing: conceptualization and measurement. *Journal of Psychology and Theology*, **11**, 330–40.

Emblen, J. D. (1992) Religion and spirituality defined according to current use in nursing literature. *Journal of Professional Nursing*, **8**(1), 41–7.

Fernsler, J., Kelman, P. and Miller, M. A. (1999) Spiritual wellbeing and demands of illness in people with colorectal cancer. *Cancer Nursing*, **22**(2), 134–40.

Fieldman, D. J. (1974) Chronic disabling illness. A holistic view. *Journal of Chronic Disability*, **22**, 287–91.

Fitchett, G. (1995) Linda Krauss and the lap of God: a spiritual assessment case study. *Second Opinion*, **20**(4), 40–9.

Fowler, J. W. (1974) Toward a developmental perspective on faith. *Religious Education*, **69**(2), 207–19.

Fry, E. (1997) Spirituality: connectedness through being and doing. In: *Spirituality: The Heart of Nursing* (ed. S. Ronaldson), pp. 5–21. Alismed Publications, Melbourne.

Granstrom, S. (1985) Spiritual care for oncology patients. *Topics in Clinical Nursing*, **7**(1), 39–45.

Gustafson, M. (1992) Prayer. In: *Independent Nursing Interventions*, 2nd edn (ed. M. Snyder), pp. 280–6. Delmar Publishers, New York.

Haase, J. E. (1987) Components of courage in chronically ill adolescents: a phenomenological study. *Advances in Nursing Science*, **9**, 64.

Hardy, A. (1979) *The Spiritual Nature of Man*. Clarendon Press, Oxford.

Hay, D. (1987) *Exploring Inner Space: Scientist and Religious Experience*. Mowbray, London.

Herth, K. and Cutcliffe, J. R. (2002) The concept of hope in nursing 3: hope and palliative care. *British Journal of Nursing*, **11**(14), 977–83.

Husserl, F. (1989) An introduction to phenomenology. In: *Introducing Philosophy: A Text with Integrated Readings*, 4th edn (ed. R. C. Solomon), pp. 268–71. Harcourt Brace, New York.

James, W. (1982) *The Varieties of Religious Experience*. Penguin, Middlesex.

Johnson, S. C. and Spilka, B. (1991) Coping with breast cancer: the roles of clergy and faith. *Journal of Religious Health*, **30**, 21–33.

Kitson, A. (1985) Spiritual care in chronic illness. In: *Nursing and Spiritual Care* (eds. O. McGilloway and F. Myco), pp. 142–55. Harper Row, London.

Kubler-Ross, E. (1975) *Death: The Final Stages of Growth*. Prentice-Hall, New Jersey.

Legere, T. (1984) A spirituality for today. *Studies in Formative Spirituality*, **5**(3), 514–20.

Lewis, K. S. (1985) *Successful Living with Chronic Illness*. Avery Publishing Group, New Jersey.

MacKinlay, E. (2001) *The Spiritual Dimension of Ageing*. Jessica Kingsley, London.

McSherry, W. (2000) *Making Sense of Spirituality in Nursing Practice*. Churchill Livingstone, Edinburgh.

Miller, J. F. (1983) *Coping with Chronic Illness*. F. A. Davies, Philadelphia.

Mische, P. (1982) Toward a global spirituality. In: *The Whole Earth Papers* (P. Mische). Global Education Association, New Jersey.

Narayanasamy, A. (1996) Spiritual care of chronically ill patients. *British Journal of Nursing*, **5**(7), 411–16.

Narayanasamy, A. (1999) A review of spirituality as applied to nursing. *International Journal of Nursing Studies*, **36**, 117–25.

Narayanasamy, A. (2000) Spiritual care and mental health competence. In: *Lyttle's Mental Health and Disorder* (eds. T. Thompson and P. Mathias), 305–24. Baillière Tindall, London.

Narayanasamy, A. (2001) *Spiritual Care: A Practical Guide for Nurses and Health Care Practitioners*, 2nd edn. Quay, Wiltshire.

Narayanasamy, A. and Owens, J. (2001) A critical incident study of nurses' responses to the spiritual needs of their patients. Journal of Advanced Nursing, **33**(4), 446–55.

Otto, R. (1950) *The Idea of the Holy*. Oxford University Press, Oxford.

Reed, P. (1992) An emerging paradigm for the investigation of spirituality in nursing. *Research in Nursing and Health*, **15**, 349–57.

Ross, L. (1997) *Nurses' Perceptions of Spiritual Care*. Aldershot, Avebury.

Sherwood, G. D. (2000) The power of nurse–client encounters. *Journal of Holistic Nursing*, **18**(2), 159–75.

Simsen, B. (1986) The spiritual dimension. *Nursing Times,* **82**(48), 41–2.

Sodestrom, K. E. and Martinson, I. M. (1987) Patients' spiritual coping strategies: a study of nurse and patient perspectives. *Oncology Nursing Forum,* **14**, 41–6.

Soeken, K. L. and Carson, V. J. (1987) Responding to the spiritual needs of the chronically ill. *Nursing Clinics of North America,* **22**(3), 603–11.

Swinton, J. (2000) *Spirituality and Mental Health Care. Rediscovering a Forgotten Dimension.* Jessica Kingsley, London.

Swinton, J. (2002) *A Space to Listen: Meeting the Spiritual Needs of People with Learning Disabilities.* The Foundation for People with Learning Disabilities, London.

Vaughan, F. (1995) *Shadows of the Sacred: Seeing Through Spiritual Illusions.* Quest Books, Wheaton.

Westerhoff, J. (1976) *Will Our Children Have Faith?* Seabury Press, New York.

Werner-Boland, B. (1980) *Grief Responses to Long-term Illness and Disability.* Prentice Hall, London.

Yates, B. C., Bensley, L. S., Lalonde, B., Lewis, F. M. and Woods, N. F. (1981) The impact of marital status and quality of family functioning in maternal chronic illness. *Health Care for Women International,* **16**, 437–49.

CHAPTER 5

A critical incident study of how nurses respond to the spiritual needs of their patients

Summary

In this chapter the findings from a critical incident study of nurses giving spiritual care are reported. Critical incidents obtained from a sample of 115 nurses working in a variety of clinical settings identified the cues that prompted spiritual care, the types of care given and the outcomes of the care. The findings suggest that there is confusion over the notion of spirituality and the role of nurses in relation to spiritual care. Interventions adopted by nurses were based on personal and intuitive experiences rather than educationally derived competencies. The approach to spiritual care was largely unsystematic and delivered in an *ad hoc* way, although there were some examples of good practice as well as areas showing scope for improvement. There was an overwhelming consensus that patients' faith and trust in nurses produces a positive effect on patients and families, and nurses themselves derived satisfaction from the experience of giving spiritual care. The study concluded that there is scope for developing an ideal model of spiritual care using the critical incident data from this study.

Key points

- Critical incidents of cues prompting spiritual care interventions and outcomes
- Spiritual, religious and cultural dimensions of care;
- Personal and intuition-based competencies; positive effects of spiritual care
- Ideal model of spiritual care interventions

Introduction

Increasingly the health care profession is calling for a more holistic approach to patient's care. With regard to this the addressing of spiritual needs is acknowledged as an essential component of holistic nursing care. In health and nursing literature holistic care is perceived as care of the body, mind and spirit (Carson, 1989; Shelley and Fish, 1988; McSherry, 2000; Shelly, 2000). There is a claim in the literature that spiritual care can be therapeutic to patients (Jourard, 1971; Millison, 1988; Morrison, 1989; Ross, 1997; Koenig, 2001).

Although empirical research on spirituality and health is developing, there is considerable literature to suggest that spiritual care is not given adequate attention in nursing. However, the phase of research related to this aspect of the role of nurses has been slow, and a fuller picture of how nurses provide spiritual care as part of a holistic care programme is yet to be established. However, much existing research is descriptive and exploratory in nature. Furthermore, these studies are short on details and fail to map out more clearly what nurses actually do when they attempt to provide spiritual care. In order to fill this gap in the research, the current study was undertaken to provide a much more comprehensive picture of how nurses construct patients' spiritual needs and provide spiritual care.

Literature review

Although nursing has its roots in spirituality, the link between these two had become less obvious when modern medicine began to make its impact on health care at the turn of the 19th century. Since the 1980s, nursing has begun to return to its traditional roots in spirituality with a steady flow of interest in the topic (Narayanasamy, 1999a), resulting in a variety of traditions and perspectives. Despite this, there is a consensus in the literature that spirituality is an important facet of humanity and that the care of body, mind and spirit is a hallmark of holistic care (Narayanasamy, 1999a; Highfields and Cason, 1983; Clifford and Gruca, 1987; Montgomery, 1991). The literature equates a state of wellbeing with the harmonious balance between these three interrelated but distinct entities: body, mind and spirit. Distress in any one of these areas affects the other, and therefore a holistic approach in restoring the harmonious balance between these three components of humanity is paramount. Research suggests that nurses are unclear about their role in providing spiritual care, but does not offer a clear picture about the precise nature of the spiritual dimensions of nursing (Ross, 1997; Harrison, 1993). The literature identifies the following barriers to spiritual care: lack of clarity among nurses as to what is spirituality, role ambiguity and lack of educational preparation for the role of spiritual care (McSherry and Draper, 1998; Ross, 1997).

There is a consensus in the nursing literature that spirituality is an elusive concept when definitions are attempted (Narayanasamy, 2000; McSherry and Draper, 1998). This problem is further compounded by the misuse of the term *spirituality*, in that this word is equated with institutional religions such as Christianity and Judaism. Several studies confirm confusion among nurses where spirituality is regarded as religion (Narayanasamy, 1993; Harrison and Burnard, 1993; Ross, 1997). According to Narayanasamy (1999b), although the UK is regarded as a secular society, the majority of nurses working in UK health care sectors have been reared in a culture permeated with Christian traditions and values. It can be inferred from this that nursing care is likely to be delivered from a value position characteristic of this Christian heritage. Some nursing theorists writing from a Christian theological perspective (Bradshaw, 1994; Shelley and Fish, 1988) are uncompromising and characterise spirituality as Christianity. However, whilst maintaining her stance on a Christian theological perspective, Bradshaw (1994), in her exposition of spirituality, does provide a comprehensive review of this subject. Others stress the universality and durability of spirituality as an everlasting phenomenon that sustains and pervades all cultures regardless of religious beliefs or non-beliefs (Hay, 1994; Macquarrie, 1972). Definitions of spirituality have been identified as:

- The essence or life principle of person (Colliton, 1981)
- A sacred journey (Mische, 1982)
- The experience of the radical truth of things (Legere, 1984)
- Giving meaning and purpose (Legere, 1984)
- A belief that relates a person to the world (Soeken and Carson, 1987)
- Being rooted in an awareness which is part of the biological make up of the human species (Narayanasamy, 1999a)

The findings of a number of studies suggest that nurses tend to perceive spiritual care as the role of the chaplains (Narayanasamy, 1993; Ross, 1997; Harrison, 1993). Ross's findings suggest that nurses who professed religious affiliation tend to attempt to provide spiritual care, but it is not clear from this study if the care given was designed to meet religious needs rather than spiritual needs. Apart from role ambiguity, factors such as lack of communication with other professionals (clergy) and environmental issues such as lack of time and space, peace, quiet and privacy interfered with nurses' attempts to provide spiritual care (Ross, 1997). The literature blames nurse education for the inadequate preparation of nurses for spiritual care in the UK (Narayanasamy, 1993; McSherry and Draper, 1999; Ross, 1997).

The findings of current research on spiritual dimensions of nursing consistently suggest that spiritual care is not given adequate attention in nursing for the three main reasons delineated above. However, much of the research reviewed so far is descriptive and exploratory in nature. Furthermore, these studies lack detail and fail to map out more clearly what nurses actually do when they attempt to provide spiritual care. In order to fill this gap in the literature, the current study was undertaken to provide a more comprehensive picture of how nurses construct patients' spiritual needs and provide spiritual care.

Aims of the study

The aims of the study are therefore to:

1. Explore how nurses respond to the spiritual needs of their patients.
2. Describe what nurses consider to be spiritual needs.
3. Typify nurses' accounts of their involvement in spiritual dimensions of care.
4. Describe the effect of nurses interventions related to spiritual care.

Methods

The nature of this study is such that a qualitative approach incorporating the critical incident technique was used. This approach is compatible with the assumptions and philosophical approaches set by Leininger (1989), Silverman (1993), Field and Morse (1985) and Flannagan (1954). The critical technique as a method of data collection was popularised by Flannagan (1954) and is particularly useful for collecting data from direct observation of human behaviour in order to facilitate problem-solving (Cormack, 1996). According to Cormack 'an incident relates to any observable human activity that is sufficiently complete in itself to permit inferences to be made' (p. 266). I decided to use this method in preference for observation because of the practical difficulties and constraints often experienced by researchers using this method. The constant presence of the researcher as an observer in the ward may interfere with nurses' roles and responsibilities to their patients. In order to avoid such problems, it was perceived by us that the aims of the current research could be achieved by the critical incident techniques. For similar reasons, Teasdale (1992) used this method for observation in his study of reassurance in nursing.

Table 5.1 Respondents' branch of nursing.

Branch of nursing	Number
Adult	85
Mental health	22
Children	8
Total	**115**

Table 5.2 Respondents' specialities.

Nursing specialities	Number
Acute adult	38
Continuing care	29
Community	18
Mental health	22
Children	8
Total	**115**

The added advantage of this method is that it depends on description of actual effective events, rather than descriptions of things as they should be. It brings credence to practice because the technique is largely concerned with the real, rather than the abstract, world and at the same time it acknowledges the constraints and limitations that we encounter in the world we live and work. Critical incidents were collected from a sample of 130 Registered Nurses working in the adult, children and mental health branches of nursing. The response rate was 88% ($n = 115$); see Tables 5.1 and 5.2.

These respondents completed questionnaires related to nursing incidents of spiritual care consisting of the following:

1. Description of a nursing situation which led up to the event; incidents; when and how nurses recognised that their patients had spiritual needs; and when this was.
2. (a) What they thought that patients' spiritual needs were.
   (b) What led them to think this.
3. Description of what they did to try to help patients to meet their spiritual needs.
4. Description of the effect on the patients/family of what they did and explanation of that conclusion.

Table 5.3 The process and outcomes of responding to patients' spiritual needs.

A. How nurses became aware of patients' spiritual needs	B. The nature of patients' reported concerns	C. The nurses' actions	D. The outcome of nurses' interventions
Religious background	Religious needs	Personal/intuitive approach, e.g. personal involvement/ engagement/ supportive	Effects on patient, e.g. feeling a sense of uniqueness and being cared for
Diagnosis-prompted	Spiritual needs	Procedural approach, e.g. logical/steps/ procedural routines	Effects on family, e.g. coming to terms/ acceptance
		Culturalist approach, e.g. honest reflexive accounts	Effects on nurses, e.g. rewarding experience
		Evangelical approach, e.g. shared religious background	

Data analysis

Data obtained from these questionnaires were subjected to content analysis. Content analysis is a flexible procedure and it enables researchers to test theoretical issues to enhance understanding of the data (Down-Wamboldt, 1992). Furthermore, this method enables data to be managed in an objective and systematic way that can lead to the drawing of inferences (Holsti, 1968). Using content analysis method, the data from the questionnaires were distilled into meaningful interpretations and these were developed to describe the findings. Initially several categories were identified and these were then collapsed into key themes related to spiritual care. These categories and themes were subjected to reviews by a panel of experts in the subject area and inter-rater validation. These measures added to the credibility of the analysis used in this research. The system of data classification (see Table 5.3) is based on the work of Cormack (1996).

Findings

How nurses became aware of the patients' spiritual needs

The description of this area is drawn exclusively from the written reports of nurses.

A majority of nurses gave accounts of incidents when they were asked how they became aware of the patients' spiritual needs. Four categories were identified in relation to this aspect of the questionnaire: *Religious background*; *Shared religious background*; *Spiritually/religiously loaded conversation*; and *Diagnosis prompted response*.

Responses comprising of any one of these factors contributed to nurses' recognition of patients concerns related to their spiritual needs. Nurses identified a variety of indicators to suggest how they recognised patients' spiritual concerns. These indicators were collapsed into the categories given above. Indicators related to these categories were included in the accounts given by nurses from all areas of nursing as identified in the methodology section. Each of these categories is described in turn.

Religious background

Nurses gave accounts that their patients' religious background suggested that they had needs in this area of their lives. Patients who stated explicitly that they belonged to a particular faith, for example, Christianity (Catholicism) prompted nurses to take measures to respond to patients' religious needs. One nurse's account reflects:

> Patient and family have strong religious needs. The patient was experiencing a psychotic illness, but wished to attend a church service each Sunday.

Likewise another nurse illustrated the following:

> A patient requested to see a priest and take confession... upset because of illness and required comfort and reassurance. Recently patient had been bereaved.

This category, religious background, was found in all areas of nursing identified in this study. The nature of the action that nurses pursued depended upon the indicators they used. Religious indicators, such as belonging to a faith (for example Christianity (Catholicism)) prompted the nurses to contact the Catholic priest at the Chaplaincy department. Such action is demonstrated in one nurse's response:

> The lady had been a practising Catholic... when she became physically ill it became apparent that she was very scared and seemed to seek comfort and began to question what was life about... she no longer wanting to worship, so didn't arrange for her to attend a service at all. I spoke with the family and following this I made arrangements for a priest to come in and give the sacraments of the sick.

Shared religious background

It seems that a number of nurses appeared to be willing to initiate spiritual care when patients shared similar religious background to them. Although fewer incidents of this nature were identified, these were significant in that such nurses built almost instant rapport with such patients. A nurse working in a ward for the care of the elderly gives an account:

> ... I was able to talk to him and reassure him. Before he died I was able to see a more relaxed person, making me feel that somehow in the end he believed some of what I was saying... I think that he was regretful of the past and was looking for a way to say sorry and to know that he would be forgiven... I told the patient that despite his past life, there is a God who cares and who promised forgiveness for those who believe and ask forgiveness...

Likewise another reflected:

> I found out that they were a Roman Catholic family... I am myself a Christian. We talked openly of our mutual faith from early on in our encounter... we prayed together.

Spiritually/religiously loaded conversation

Further analysis of nurses' accounts suggests that spiritually/religiously loaded conversation with patients and their families prompted them to initiate actions to meet their patients' needs. Nurses identified a number of indicators related to this aspect of patients'/relatives' conversation. These indicators were collapsed into the above category. The following quotes from nurses' accounts suggest the basis for nurses' actions related to spiritual care intervention. One nurse's account demonstrates spiritually loaded conversation:

> On a psychiatric ward, I used to spend considerable time talking with this patient. His spiritual needs seemed to be just to talk about what he believed, what he doubted and somewhere to find hope and strength, something to be angry with...

Likewise, another nurse gives the following picture:

> A clinic situation in which the patient was told that she had metastatic disease that would not respond to curative treatment... experienced loss of hope leading to despair and she was desperate to have something to fill the vacuum in her life. I felt this was the point when her spiritual needs were identified

Nurses' accounts representing the above category featured in all of the areas identified in this study.

Diagnosis prompted response

A number of nurses responded to patients' diagnoses as indicators of spiritual needs. Some nurses resorted to a variety of spiritual care interventions to reassure patient and relatives. One nurse responded to a patient's diagnosis as follows:

> The situation occurred when a patient wanted to know his diagnosis – no medical staff was available, and it was felt that a member of staff he knew rather than a doctor he didn't know would be more appropriate as the bearer of bad news. He had carcinoma of the lung... being aware of his strong Christian beliefs I was only made aware of this when he asked if I would object to saying a prayer.... At the time I felt reassurance and support in a time of crisis was his need – to communicate his distress without distressing his family.

Another nurse working on a continuing care ward recalls:

> One lady admitted to the ward was a Mormon, although religion is only a part of spirituality, for this lady it was a very essential part of her expression of her spirituality. She was very keen to be able to practise her beliefs and religion whilst hospitalised. It was during the assessment on admission that this was the case. For many patients the hospital can

provide opportunity to practice religions and enable them to maintain this aspect of their spirituality. But it was appreciated that here was a case where a lady had openly expressed her need to practice, but difficult to meet this on the ward with no hospital provision for Mormons.

According to the critical incidents provided by nurses from the various areas of nursing most of them initiated action that attempted to address the spiritual needs of their patients. However, as in the example above, there were fewer instances where nurses were unable to initiate spiritual care interventions for lack of provision for meeting the needs of patients from less popular faiths.

The nature of patients' reported concerns

With respect to this aspect of the questionnaire respondents gave accounts which were categorised into two areas: religious needs and spiritual needs. Each of these categories produced several sub-categories. These are identified and described below.

Religious needs

Religious beliefs

Many nurses gave accounts that suggest that nurses interpreted many patients' spiritual concerns in terms of religious beliefs. As suggested in the previous section, indicators related to religious beliefs prompted a large number of incidents of interventions that could be described as religious care. One nurse's account suggests this:

> The nursing team as a whole recognised towards the latter stage of patients' life that he became very aggressive and hostile. His relatives felt that this was due to lack of attention to his spiritual needs, and they admitted that patient had been deeply religious until tragic events took over.... It took time for the nursing team to sit with the family and patient to work out what was required, which led to eventual pastoral support.

Another nurse from a medical ward gave this account:

> I was nursing a patient with an end stage chronic illness, who was difficult to communicate with, appeared quite angry about his situation....

I had no idea what his needs were, I felt frustrated by being unable to help him with his inability to accept his illness. I was relieved when his family suggested contacting the minister.... I realised something was wrong as they were quite angry but not really aware what it was initially.... Following a long talk with his minister patient became more settled and accepting of his illness and imminent death.

Across all areas of nursing, respondents gave accounts of incidents that suggest that patients with religious beliefs appear to prompt them to initiate spiritual care that could be described as religious in nature. Needs identified as religious are often referred to the chaplains to visit patients.

Religious practices

Some of the reported concerns can be described as to do with religious practices. Many nurses felt that in clearly stated concerns related to religious practices such as prayer, attending mass, church services, receiving the Holy Communion, last rites etc., nurses appear to be responding to such needs. In many cases it is patients' relatives who reminded nurses to initiate such actions.
One nurse recalls the importance of religious practices for a patient:

I nursed an elderly patient who had been a missionary for most of his life.... He needed to maintain his previous lifestyle... needed to carry on attending mass....

Another nurse mentions a patient requiring last rites:

A patient was a practising Catholic, his condition deteriorated considerably... family informed me that patient would want last rites... I phoned the Chaplain who came in to perform last rites during the night.

Symbolic

Apart from religious practices, participants in this study gave accounts of symbolic aspects of patients' spiritual concerns. A nurse gives an account that illustrates the symbolic nature of her spiritual concerns:

This patient arrived on to the ward very ill. I knew her death was imminent. This patient was still able to communicate minimally with non-verbal communication.... Her spiritual need in this case was a religious one... she wanted to die in peace. As I was washing her she reached for her necklace, it was her Cross. I admired her for her faith in the Cross, that was her comfort.

Similarly, a nurse working in the mental health area recalls:

An elderly lady admitted for self neglect with Irish background, was devotedly Catholic and had the Crucifix and statues, etc.... We had a great understanding of her faith... we managed to contact her priest, who was very supportive of both patient and staff.... She appeared to get a great deal of satisfaction and release from having her priest around her....

Another nurse gave an account that reflected similar features;

This patient appeared to take comfort and solace from not only being able to attend a church service but also from having religious artefacts in her room. These were brought into hospital by her family. She expressed that to be in communion with God gave her strength to cope with her illness.

Accounts of the symbolic nature of patients' concerns were reported by nurses across all areas of nursing identified in this study.

Spiritual needs

A number of nurses identified patients' spiritual concerns in non-religious terms, which included: expression of feelings/emotions; sources of strength; love and relatedness; meaning and purpose; and peace/tranquillity. An analysis of these follows next.

Expression of feelings/emotions

Several nurses gave accounts of incidents of expression of feelings/emotions which they considered to be spiritual concerns. These were identified as indicators that suggested that something was wrong with patients which prompted them to initiate actions that attempted to meet spiritual needs. One nurse recalls an incident related to this:

Through our conversation, fear became the overriding factor causing tense and emotional pain. Patient was afraid of dying and didn't want to upset her husband in relaying her fears.

Another nurse working in the community gave a similar account:

> I allowed the patient to express his thoughts about how he felt – what his beliefs were and although I didn't feel I had the religious knowledge I felt able to listen...

Some nurses described incidents in which patients sought or derived sources of strength that gave them spiritual comfort as a coping mechanism with regard to their illness. The above nurse added:

> I was nursing a dying patient – he had a real need to talk to about God and to 'confess' deeds in the past. It seemed quite appropriate to contact the local minister to visit. This provided patient with comfort and an ear and a 'confession of his past'. Afterwards he seemed to be more able to come to terms with his impending death and his family seemed less stressed out with the situation at home.

Meaning and purpose

According to some nurses their patients' spiritual needs manifested as a search for meaning and purpose. Some patients appeared to be struggling to find meaning and purpose as result of illness. Critical points in life such as the diagnosis of cancer and other terminal illnesses prompted patients to search for meaning and purpose. An oncology nurse's account suggests this:

> A patient needed guidance, seeking meaning and purpose... wanting someone to guide him through his emotional turmoil.... I tried to talk to the patient and his family but I felt out of depth and asked them to speak to a more experienced colleague.... I didn't feel I had enough knowledge or confidence to completely guide them through [the] situation.

In contrast, a nurse working in medical care appear to be capable of dealing with patients' spiritual concerns:

> A patient wanted to talk to nurses about seriousness of illness and seek answers... issues 'concerning life' and 'why her'.... I tried to be honest as possible and discuss the thoughts and feelings of 'meaning of life and 'why her' to a degree that I felt comfortable with.

The nurses' action

Nurses' accounts of their actions related to spiritual care suggest that they adopted certain strategies when spiritual needs were identified. Personal experience, beliefs, practice culture, and personal and professional knowledge influenced the type of strategies they used. These strategies are broadly categorised as follows: *personal/intuitive approach*; *procedural approach*; *culturalist approach*; and *evangelical approach*. Each of these strategies is identified and described in turn.

Personal/intuitive approach

Nurses' accounts suggest that some of them used a personal/intuitive approach. Nurses who used this approach appear to be highly intuitive and sensitive in recognising needs which could be described as spiritual in nature. They responded to the affective dimensions of patients' needs such as expressions of feelings/emotions. They were willing to immerse fully in all aspects of their patients' care. This led to the formation of relationships with patients and relatives on equal terms with an emphasis on partnership. Nurses adopting this approach used counselling as a strategy for reassurance. They showed extreme levels of understanding and sensitivity when addressing patients' spiritual needs. In the analysis further sub-categories were added to the main personal/intuitive approach category to illustrate this strategy. Extracts from nurses' accounts are given to support these sub-categories as follows:

Personal involvement/engagement/supportive

Nurses' accounts suggest that those who adopted the personal/intuitive approach often had detailed knowledge about their patients. They were willing to be personally involved and engaged in all aspects of their patients' care. They were extremely supportive of patients and their family. These nurses described their experience as rewarding (see next section). A nurse working in a medical ward recalls:

> I tried to be as honest as possible and discuss the thoughts and feelings of 'meaning of life and 'why her' to a degree that I felt comfortable with.... I feel that the patient and family appreciated 'honest' answers, and grew to trust the staff as we didn't make any 'false' promises. I think this because they seemed to feel at ease to discuss their most intimate

thoughts and feelings until they took their mother home to die. By the time they did this they appeared to all (including the patient) accept that death was inevitable.

Partnership/symmetrical relationship

Nurses who used the personal/intuitive approach portrayed a nurse–patient relationship that could be regarded as a symmetrical one. Nurses, patients and their relatives became partners in the suffering, experience and care. One nurse's account illustrates this:

> This patient was an American lady on holiday here, came as an emergency when she had an extended M.I. She was transferred to us, she related well to me... she wanted a visit from the priest. This expressed how she felt and wanted to make peace with God, I took her to the chapel to pray. After this the chaplain visited her on the ward... from then on she began to speak openly about her religious needs and her closeness to her family.

Nurses who used the personal/intuitive approach helped patients to cope with their illness and suffering. They supported patients to find meaning in life and suffering.

Counselling

Many nurses adopting the personal/intuitive approach used counselling as a way of helping patients to cope with their illness and supported them throughout their time in hospital. Because of their ability to be intuitive and sensitive they used counselling instantly as soon as they realised that something was spiritually wrong with their patients. One nurse's account illustrates this:

> The patient was a young driver involved in an RTA where her passenger, her mother was killed.... I spent three hours with her to help to try to come terms with this as she blamed herself. I reassured her and gave her the time and space... she became gradually calmer and seemed to accept that the accident was not her fault... finally I referred her to the bereavement counsellor...

Nurses using the personal/intuitive approach provided reassurance to patients and relatives through counselling with beneficial effects to all parties.

Procedural approach

Almost all nurses who equated religious needs with spiritual needs adopted a procedural approach to spiritual care. Within this approach a range of features were identified and given sub-categories in the analysis. These sub-categories are described in the context of nurses' accounts as follows.

Responding to religious needs

Several nurses responded to the religious needs of patients in terms of indicators discussed earlier. Patients identified as religious or as belonging to particular faiths were seen as having religious needs. Many of the patients with religious as opposed to spiritual needs were almost immediately referred to the Chaplaincy department. In this respect Christian patients (Catholics) were more frequently referred to the priests for religious care and rituals. An extract from a nurse's account illustrates this well:

> On admission of the patient it was apparent that the patient was Church of England and went to church every Sunday. They spoke openly about their religious beliefs and used the church with health problems to combat illness in the past. The patient had a Myocardial Infarction and on initial assessment were asked if they would like to go to church when well they were in favour of this.... I felt that the patient would like to see the Chaplain in the hospital when well enough to go but that the patient may appreciate him at the bedside. I was able to confirm this as the patient was so grateful when I proposed the idea.

Logical steps/procedural routines

Most of the nurses who identified patients as having religious needs took logical steps and adhered to procedural routines too as an attempt to meet their religious needs. At times the approach was done to a precision which could be described as an 'Open and shut case' approach. This approach appeared to be prevalent among nurses working in medical and surgical settings. Some of the nurses' accounts demonstrate this approach.

> The family alerted nurses to the fact that the patient was religious and would like a visit from their priest. I arranged for the priest to visit. I

gave privacy for them and ensured that the family were aware of this visit

Controlling and regulatory

A number of nurses who used a logical and procedural routine and tend to use language and metaphors could be characterised as controlling and regulatory in practice. One nurse gives an account that portrays the controlling and regulatory approach to spiritual care.

> An elderly lady admitted for self neglect with Irish origins... she was a Catholic... a devout Catholic and had the crucifix and statues.... It is policy of the unit to allow all patients access to spiritual help and as such we contacted the local priest...

Some of the nurses who used the procedural approach not only appeared to be controlling and regulatory but adopted a relationship which could be described as asymmetrical and impersonal in nature. In some situations nurses remained uninvolved, but ensured that routines were followed without being a participant in the patient's spiritual care.

Stereotyping

Some nurses using the procedural approach were typifying patients into stereotypes in terms of cultural and religious backgrounds. Patients identified as from a particular culture or religion were subjected to certain routines. For example, an account from a nurse working in the mental health field illustrates this:

> We had a lady who was a Muslim.... I spoke to her partner in order to get some insight into this faith. I explained to her that we could get in touch with someone from the community if needed.

Culturalist approach

A number of nurses gave accounts of incidents related to spiritual care which suggests that they had adopted an approach that could be described as culturalistic in nature. In this approach nurses appear to be sensitive to the cultural and religious background of patients. They gave specific consideration to the cultural and religious needs of their patients. With this approach several sub-categories were identified in the analysis. These are identified and described below.

Symbolic interactionism

The cultural and religious identity of patients and related factors provided symbolic cues for some nurses to be sensitive in their approach to them. They made efforts to find out from patients and their relatives information that could best help them to provide care that takes into consideration the cultural and religious needs of their patients. These included patients from cultural and religious groups such as Muslims from Middle Eastern and south Asian backgrounds and Hindus from an Indian sub-continent background. Some of the nurses' accounts suggest that they not only appeared to be sensitive to patients' cultural and religious needs but they remained committed to cultural and religious care.

> Clients who wish to pray to Mecca may have the curtains pulled round, be given a side ward or taken to the mosque on D floor as does happen... cutstoms of different cultures/religions are recognised as they arise and every effort made to accommodate requests

Honest reflexivity

Some of the nurses' accounts gave the impression that although they were committed to cultural care, they felt that organisational constraints, lack of policies, support from colleagues and poor knowledge led to frustrations that needs are not being met adequately. A nurse working in the community reflected:

> Some family members needed more support than others, although with a young family I felt it was hard enough coping with them, work, and my own emotions to try to meet their spiritual needs.

Another nurse working in medical ward reflected:

> I realised something was wrong as they were quite angry but not really aware what it was.... All I feel I did was contact the minister at the patient's request. I did try to speak to the patient, but as my beliefs were not as strong as theirs, felt I was of little comfort to them.

Evangelical approach

A few nurses used an approach that could be typified as evangelical in nature. Several sub-categories emerged from nurses' accounts related to the evangelical approach. These are identified and described below.

Shared background

These nurses felt at ease when they realised that patients shared a similar religious background with them. Christian nurses in particular, when they realised that patients shared a similar faith, used this as a common platform to establish a firm nurse–patient relationship. Some felt comfortable with initiating religious care.

> We both shared similar religious beliefs. I think he was regretful of the past and was looking for a way to say sorry and to know that he would be forgiven.... I told the patient despite his past life that there is a God who cares and who promised forgiveness for those who believe and who ask for forgiveness.

Imposing

Some nurses appeared determined to impose their personal beliefs, although they used indirect means to achieve these. When opportunities arose they used them to impose their personal beliefs upon patients and their families.

> A baby was critically ill on Christmas Eve... baby had not been baptised, I suggested to the parents that they may be would like to talk to a chaplain... the mother declined but the Dad wanted to, so I contacted a chaplain who came to talk to them... the mother was adamant that she did not want her baby baptised... I suppose my personal beliefs and... motivated me to take this action. The chaplain arrived, the mum changed her mind. The baby was baptised with myself present. I felt this helped the parents immensely.

The outcome of the nurses' interventions

The outcome of the nurses' interventions had effects on patients, their families and nurses. Many descriptors of the effects of nurses' interventions were identified in the analysis from their accounts. These are described below.

Becoming relaxed, peaceful and calmer

Many nurses commented that spiritual care interventions enable patients to become relaxed, peaceful and calmer. Both types of intervention, spiritual and religious care, result in similar types of effect. A nurse working in the mental health field reflected:

> ... by explaining and showing him about the need to think of the future, he was able to see that there was something beyond the here and now, which made him more relaxed and comfortable... he became more relaxed and less fearful. The expression on his face said it all.

Feeling comforted and supported

Some nurses gave accounts of their spiritual care interventions where patients felt comforted and supported. One nurse's account demonstrates this:

> My action brought them together, they felt comforted and supported... it gave them some control

Expression of gratitude

Nurses gave accounts that their interventions brought about positive outcomes. One nurse reflected:

> I was there when patient needed me and I did not try to make it any less profound than it was.... She was grateful.

Another recalled:

> The family were satisfied that they had carried out the correct procedure and thanked us for our support.

Feeling a sense of uniqueness and being cared for

Some nurses suggested that spiritual care interventions had positive effects on patients where they derived a sense of uniqueness and being cared for. A nurse working in the mental health field recounts:

> On a psychiatric ward I used to spend considerable time talking with this patient.... Sometimes he would ask if I could read a particular passage to him or listen to him singing or sit with him praying. This we did together. I never challenged his beliefs but accepted them and tried to be just there.... I believe the effect of this was that it helped this patient to explore areas of his life he was having problems with. It helped him to feel, at least in the short-term, someone cared....

Feeling stronger to cope

A few nurses suggested that their spiritual care interventions enable patients to derive a sense of security in which they felt stronger to cope with their illness and problems. One nurse reflected:

> My intervention gave the patient the opportunity to fully vent his feelings and fears. By addressing his fears in a supportive environment I felt he was left in a stronger position to cope.

Effects on family

Many nurses recalled that their spiritual care interventions had positive effects on patients' families. Many expressed gratitude, feeling comforted and happy and coming to terms/accepting of the situation related to their relative's illness. Some of the nurses' accounts are categorised as follows.

Expression of gratitude

> She wished to die in a situation which was familiar to her and according to her beliefs and family history. I put a mattress on the floor and did all her care there.... The family were grateful for this, even though they found it a bit embarrassing.

Feeling comforted and happy

> ... patient and family were pleased that we attempted to fulfil their needs and thanked us because they felt happy and comforted.

Coming to terms/acceptance

> Following a long talk with his minister patient became more settled and accepting of his illness and imminent death... by being able to speak to the minister again, I feel the minister was able to comfort the patient and enable him and his family to accept things. The patient became more happy ... felt able to cope...

Effects on nurses

Many nurses felt that giving spiritual care has been a rewarding experience. Some expressed that they derived great satisfaction from this role. However, others felt spiritual care interventions posed ethical dilemmas for them. Some of these accounts are as follows.

Rewarding experience

One nurse reflected with colleagues that things went well:

> The relationships forged seemed to have quite strong bonds in particular with a small group of nurses.... Patient and family felt special recognising the effort staff showed to understand their specific circumstances and beliefs... led to the conclusion through positive feedback from patients and families, as well as intuition and reflection with colleagues that things went well.

Ethical dilemma

> The patient was admitted to the ward with lower back pain and abnormal Hb... he wished to put his life in order after being told the diagnosis. He also refused to see the chaplain but wished to speak to particular

members of staff... the patient discussed his feelings of satisfaction surrounding his wedding and the last few days of his life. He felt he could face death knowing he had made provision for his family.... His family, especially his new wife, were more difficult to assess than the care we had given for them. It is frustrating that here there is no way to follow the bereaved through.

Discussion

The themes and categories that emerged from the critical incidents data and the emerging theoretical understanding derived from the analysis are described and discussed below (see Table 5.3). The subcategories related to the main categories are given in bold and italic type.

Nurses' awareness of patients' spiritual needs

The findings of this study suggested that nurses in the course of their encounters with patients became aware of patients' spiritual needs when the following were recognised: patients' religious background, shared religious background, spiritually/religiously loaded conversation and diagnosis. These acted as strong prompters for nurses to respond to their patients' spiritual needs.

Religious background

Information about patients' religious background acted as a strong indicator for nurses to initiate action that brought about religious care interventions. This background information offered a concrete means to deliver services that could be described as religious in nature rather than spiritual. The Chaplaincy services were used frequently as a way of meeting patients' perceived religious needs.

Shared religious background

Besides identification of patients' religious needs, when nurses knew that patients shared a similar religious background with them they felt this offered them the opportunity to develop a close relationship with the patient. Such status legitimised their interventions related to spiritual care. Ross (1997) identified in her study that nurses who claimed religious affiliation were better than those without in identifying patients' spiritual needs. It can be inferred from this claim that nurses' personal belief systems influenced their participation in spiritual care. This is consistent with the findings of other studies, where the link between nurses' willingness to be involved in general and spiritual care and their personal belief system has been established (Forrest, 1989; Samarel, 1991; Piles, 1986).

Spiritual/religious loaded conversation

When patients' conversation was found to have strong spiritual/religious dimensions nurses used these as prompters to initiate spiritual care interventions. Nurses who used a personal approach often picked up cues which could be described as spiritual in nature to initiate spiritual care interventions. This suggests that nurses who used a personal approach are more responsive to patients' spiritual needs as opposed to religious needs. This is consistent with Ross's (1997) findings, where she found that nurses who demonstrated personal characteristics of this nature gave spiritual care at a deeper level than those lacking them. Where needs were identified as religious in nature these were referred to hospital chaplains or other religious experts.

Diagnosis-prompted response

Apart from religious needs and shared background, patients' diagnoses acted as a strong prompter for nurses to initiate spiritual care interventions. The severity of the diagnosis often prompted nurses to initiate interventions to meet patients' spiritual needs. Cancer and other forms of terminal illness prompted nurses to give 'on the spot' spiritual care and in some instances the hospital chaplains were called to supplement the nurses' efforts and to provide 'expert' help.

The nature of patients' reported concerns

Religious needs

Nurses' reported concerns centred around two areas which could be described as religious needs and spiritual needs in broad terms. Expression of *religious beliefs and practices* led nurses to initiate religious care interventions. In many instances these needs were referred to the chaplains who were called to see patients. On some occasions, in response to reported concerns nurses prayed with patients or encouraged them to carry out religious practices and rituals. In particular, the wishes of patients from ethnic minority backgrounds were respected and considered sensitively. For example, dietary needs related to the patient's religion and culture were considered as part of the care planning. Similar considerations were given in the case of dying patients who were from minority cultural and religious groups.

The symbolic aspects of some patients' lives, such as the cross, crucifix and religious artefacts, acted as concrete factors that led to recognition of religious needs and these prompted nursing attention.

It appears that nurses were good at recognising religious needs in terms of the above factors. In almost all cases religious care interventions took place when such factors were identified. Although this is a good sign, it may be the case that other spiritual needs, such as the search for meaning and purpose and the need for love and security, could have been overlooked. The literature considers these factors to be an important part of patients' spiritual dimension (Narayanasamy, 1999b; Legere, 1984). There is consensus in the literature that although nurses usually display some knowledge of and ability to identify the concrete aspects of patients' religious needs, for example communion (Ross, 1997; Narayanasamy, 1993; Chadwick, 1973), they find it more difficult to recognise spiritual needs, those which could be described as predominantly psychological in nature (Highfields and Cason, 1983).

Spiritual needs

This finding in the current study showed an indication of change in that a number of nurses identified patients' spiritual concerns in non-religious terms, which included *expressions of feelings/emotions*, and *searching for meaning and purpose*.

Nurses in this study who used a more personal approach that allowed them to identify emotional tensions and turmoil made efforts to be involved in giving counselling support to patients to overcome their spiritual distress. This is consistent with Ross's study, in which she found nurses who had clear views about the meaning of life and wider issues often engaged at a deeper level with patients when providing spiritual care.

The nurses' action

The findings of this study suggest that nurses, on identification of patients' spiritual/religious needs, used four approaches: personal, procedural, culturalist, and evangelical. These will be discussed in turn.

Personal approach

Many nurses who described spiritual needs in non-religious terms tended to use a more personal approach. These needs related to emotional feelings, thoughts and expression of the need to explore meaning and purpose by patients.

Nurses who adopted this approach were giving a lot of attention to patients. They were also engaged in all aspects of patient care. This approach to spiritual care could be described as holistic. The relationship with patients tended to be **mutual** and based on an equal **partnership** that prompted feelings of trust and security among patients. Nurses used a **counselling** approach and often supported patients during critical stages of their **illness**. The findings of this aspect of the study are consistent with the literature, which stresses the importance of a personal approach comprising of the elements identified earlier (Montgomery 1991). Montgomery (1991), in her study of 'the care-giving relationship, paradoxical and transcendent aspects', observes that nurses who allow themselves to be close to patients actually experience, on some level, the patient's healing, or the positive effects of their caring. It would seem that this approach could be considered to be the ideal model for spiritual care.

Procedural approach

The procedural approach tended to address needs which could be described as religious in nature. Patients' expression of *religious beliefs and practices* are perceived as spiritual needs. Nurses in the study who used this approach took *logical steps* and adhered to *procedural routines* when addressing patients' religious needs. Many who used this approach referred patients to the chaplains to visit them on the ward. *Stereotyping* of patients in terms of religious and cultural labels was common among nurses in this study who followed the procedural approach. Some nurses who used this approach appeared to be addressing patients' religious needs as a way of appeasing relatives rather than meeting patients' wishes. Nurses sometimes colluded and collaborated with patients' families, often without patients' prior knowledge, before initiating action directly or indirectly related to spiritual/religious care interventions.

Although the procedural approach is commendable in addressing the religious and cultural needs of patients, nurses often appeared to be impersonal in their approach in that procedures and religious routines set the tone for spiritual care intervention. This state of practice raises the question of whether spiritual distress displayed in non-religious terms and expressions would receive any spiritual care interventions from nurses. It may be that such expressions would go unnoticed. Stereotyping of patients in terms of religious and cultural needs may lead to rigid application of religious practices and routines without consideration of actual needs related to patients' spirituality. Concerns are expressed in the literature that certain groups of people may be treated in a rigid way in terms of assumptions about their race, culture and faiths.

Such an approach also raises the possibility that nurses feel secure in adhering to concrete mechanical means to deal with patients' spiritual/religious needs. It is also likely that a nursing culture based on doing things for patients in terms of concrete and tangible measures lends itself well to the procedural approach. The high incidence of referral to the chaplains to deal with patients' religious needs may be part of this picture, and such measures may have acted as a shield to respondents' perceived inadequacies in spiritual care knowledge and competencies. This aspect of the finding is consistent with Narayanasamy's (1993) study, which found that nurses depended on religious agents such as the hospital chaplains to shield them from getting involved in spiritual care due to their poor knowledge and skills related to spiritual care. In a similar vein, Millison (1988) suggests that many carers steer clear of spiritual care for lack of skill in this area or because they simply feel that it is not part of their role.

Culturalist approach

A small number of nurses in this study used a cultural interactionist approach to initiate spiritual care interventions. Patients perceived to be belonging to minority faiths and cultures were recognised with relative ease by nurses.

Patients' cultural and religious identities gave nurses vital clues about what course of action was to be initiated to meet these needs. Nurses using this approach took a holistic approach in which they consulted and involved relatives and families to be part of the overall care. Participants sought expert advice as well in addressing the cultural and spiritual needs of patients belonging to minority cultural and religious groups. These nurses took practical measures to ensure that privacy and special provisions were available to these groups of patients where feasible. However, when they were unable to make special provisions for patients from minority religious and cultural groups they gave ***honest reflexive*** accounts of why they failed to measure up to expectations of good spiritual and cultural care.

These shortcomings were due to lack of support from colleagues and lack of practical provisions to meet such needs. The inability to be comprehensive in their approach led to ethical dilemmas for these nurses, feeling that they could provide better care if they had adequate knowledge, skills, peer and management support, and resources. The ethical principles of beneficence and justice as described by Beauchamp and Childress (1994) have the potential to be compromised.

Evangelical approach

A small number of nurses gave accounts of spiritual care incidents which could be described as using an evangelical approach. Nurses who **shared a similar religious background** with patients made great efforts to reaffirm patients' faith, especially if they appeared to be relapsed Christians.

Likewise, in the case of very ill babies and infants some nurses in this study went out of their way to baptise them in order to fulfil their own religious beliefs. When opportunities arose they used them to impose their personal beliefs upon patients and their families. Although these nurses avoided direct coercion, they were very persuasive in encouraging parents to consider baptism for their babies and infants. Nurses gave several incidents related to outcomes of success with their persuasion. Some nurses believed that baptism actually saved some children from death as a result of serious illness. These religious convictions and subsequent evangelical approach seemed to be prompted by a belief in Divine interventions when medical care was failing.

However well intended the evangelical approach is, it raises ethical questions. Although the numbers were small it is likely that this study may have reflected a larger problem with regard to evangelism within nursing. However, it could be argued, as Benson and Stark (1996) put it, that if such measures do not produce harm as it conforms to the principles of non-maleficence (Beauchamp and Childress, 1994), then there is no problem. Likewise, the principles of autonomy (Beauchamp and Childress, 1994) have been followed in that patients/parents have fully consented to nurses' actions, although autonomy and consent in an unequal power relationship (health care worker and patient) could be questioned. In spite of these claims, such nursing actions could be perceived as unacceptable practices from an ethical point of view in terms of the imposition of personal values on a vulnerable group of individuals.

The outcome of the nurses' interventions

Nurses from this study identified that the outcome of their spiritual care interventions had therapeutic effects on patients, families and nurses on most occasions.

Positive effect on patients and relatives

Following spiritual care interventions, patients appeared **peaceful, relaxed and calm, and grateful**. Such states would aid patients' healing and recovery (or peaceful death). Added to this, nurses in this study reported that many patients felt **comforted and supported** as a direct result of spiritual care interventions. Some patients reported that they derived **a sense of feeling unique and cared for**, while others **felt stronger to cope** as a direct outcome of spiritual care intervention. From this it could be surmised that spiritual care interventions, directly or indirectly, reduced distress and enabled patients to gather emotional strength to cope with their illness and suffering. It can be assumed that indicators of spiritual wellbeing could be developed using these descriptors. Presently, indicators of spiritual wellbeing based on empirical evidence are not readily available. The descriptors related to spiritual wellbeing could be used for the development of spiritual care indicators when evaluation of spiritual care is being considered.

Effects on family

Further to the above effects of spiritual care interventions on patients, nurses gave accounts which suggested that such interventions had positive effects on patients' families as well. Many families expressed *gratitude* and *feelings of being comforted and happy* as a result of spiritual care interventions by nurses. In addition to this effect, some relatives *came to terms* with patients' illness by *accepting* the situation. This general state of wellbeing of patients and families is a product of holistic care, of which spiritual care is an important dimension.

Effects on nurses

Apart from patients and relatives, nurses from this study gave accounts that suggest that they felt that giving spiritual care and the effects it had on patients was a *rewarding experience*.

This suggests that nurses' personal involvement by being supportive of patients during distress and being able to give time and attention to patients' spiritual needs is rewarding. There is probably a strong link between the personal approach to spiritual care and the rewarding experience felt by nurses, although almost all nurses in this study suggested that they derived a positive effect from this. This part of the study provides strong evidence that spiritual care should be an integral part of the nurse's role, as it can be a rewarding experience. The significance of this experience should be emphasised in nurse education and training programmes on spiritual care. Tentatively, it could be suggested that if spiritual care is an active component of a nurse's role it is most likely to be rewarding and satisfying, leading to overall improved role satisfaction and morale among nurses.

However, some nurses from this study gave accounts that suggested that the inability to provide proper spiritual care due to lack of peer and management support, poor training and education and resources, posed *ethical dilemmas*. These nurses gave honest reflexive accounts in which they expressed that they felt unfulfilled as they intuitively felt that they were unable to help patients with their spiritual needs.

However, the overall finding adds strength to the earlier claim that spiritual care interventions lead to positive outcomes in patients and relatives, and this state of practice has further effects on nurses where they equally derived a sense of fulfilment. Messages of this nature derived from empirical evidence should be disseminated to all nurses and health care managers.

Limitations of the study

This study could have been followed up by further interviews with nurses to establish comparability between written and oral accounts of incidents related to spiritual care. The sample size from the children and mental health branches of nursing could have been expanded to elicit more incidents of spiritual care. Therefore caution is needed when generalisation is being considered from the findings of this study, given the small sample size from these two branches of nursing. Although the data analysis was subjected to reviews by a panel of experts in the subject area and inter-rater validation, there is still a danger that the researchers' bias and values may have influenced interpretations. The other limitation is that this study does not include samples from the learning disability nursing branch. However, in spite of these limitations the strength of this study lies in its ecological validity, in that it is based on real accounts from nurse respondents working in a variety of clinical settings. Overall, this study provides scope for more research involving in-depth interviews to follow up some of the issues which could benefit from further exploration.

Conclusion

This research is the first of its kind in the study of spiritual care as described by nurse participants. Overall, the findings suggest that there is confusion over the notion of spirituality and roles related to spiritual care. A variety of models of spiritual care emerged in this study from the critical incidents derived from nurse respondents. These models of care are very much based on personal and intuitive experiences rather than educationally derived competencies. Therefore it appears that the approach to spiritual care is unsystematic and delivered in an *ad hoc* way, although there were some good examples of practice as well as areas showing scope for improvement. Whatever the approaches are, there appears to be an overwhelming consensus that faith and trust in nurses produce a positive effect on patients and families. This is consistent with Benson and Stark's (1996) work, in which they demonstrated a clear link between positive nurse–patient relationships and healing. Likewise, Montgomery (1991) suggests nurses' closeness to patients and willingness to share their experiences have a positive effect and promote healing. This adds weight to the claim that there is a close link between the body, mind and spirit. A harmonious balance between these three elements is paramount for the wellbeing of patients. The findings of the study suggest that nurse participants also derived satisfaction when they implemented spiritual care. In this respect, spiritual care interventions promote mostly a sense of wellbeing in nurses as well.

The findings of this study offer prospects for developing the personal and cultural approaches of care as models of spiritual care. The elements of good practices from both approaches can be drawn together to produce a model of spiritual care that could be piloted and tested for validation. The unintended outcome of this study is that it produced 115 incidents of spiritual care that could be used as vignettes for problem-solving teaching related to spiritual care. It is hoped that this will be the basis for our next research project: to develop an ideal model of spiritual care using the rich data derived from this study.

Acknowledgements

This study is a larger part of a project on spiritual care research sponsored by Trinity Care plc. We would like to thank the nurses who participated in this study.

An adapted version of this report is published in Narayanasamy, A. and Owen, J. (2001) A critical incident study of nurses' responses to the spiritual needs of their patients. *Journal of Advanced Nursing*, **33**(4), 446–55.

References

Bradshaw, A. (1994) *Lighting the Lamp: The Spiritual Dimension of Nursing Care*. Scutari Press, London.

Benson, H. with Stark, M. (1996) *Timeless Healing: Power and Biology of Belief.* Simon & Schuster, London.

Beauchamp, T. L. and Childress, J. F. (1994) *Principles of Biomedical Ethics,* 4th edn). Oxford University Press, New Jersey.

Carson, V. B. (1989) *Spiritual Dimensions of Nursing Practice.* W. B. Saunders Company, Philadelphia.

Chadwick, R. (1973) Awareness and preparedness of nurses to meet spiritual needs. *The Nurse's Lamp,* **22**(6), 2–8.

Clifford, B. S. and Gruca, J. A. (1987) Facilitating spiritual care in rehabilitation. *Rehabilitation Nursing,* **12**(6), 331–3.

Colliton, M. (1981) The spiritual dimension of nursing. In: *Clinical Nursing* (eds. E. Belland and J. Y. Passos). Macmillan, New York.

Cormack, D. (1996) *The Research Process in Nursing,* 3rd edn. Blackwell, Oxford.

Down-Wamboldt, B. (1992) Content analysis-method, application and issue. *Health Care for Women International,* **13**(3), 313–21.

Field, P. A. and Morse, J. (1985) *Nursing Research, the Application of Qualitative Approaches.* Chapman & Hall, London.

Flannagan, J. C. (1954) The critical incident technique. *Psychological Bulletin,* **51**(4), 327–58.

Forrest, D. (1989) The experience of caring. *Journal of Advanced Nursing,* **14**(14), 815–23.

Harrison, J. (1993) Spirituality and nursing practice. *Journal of Clinical Nursing,* **2**, 211–17.

Harrison, J. and Burnard, P. (1993) *Spirituality and Nursing Practice.* Avebury, Aldershot.

Hay, D. (1994) On the biology of God: what is the current status of Hardy's Hypothesis? *International Journal for the Psychology of Religion,* **4**(1), 1–23.

Highfields, M. F. and Cason, C. (1983) Spiritual needs of patients: are they recognised? *Cancer Nursing,* June, 187–92.

Holsti, O. R. (1968) Content analysis. In: *The Hand Book of Social Psychology,* Vol. 2 (eds. G. Lindsay and E. Aronson). Addison-Wesley, Reading.

Jourard, S. (1971) *The Transparent Self.* Van Nostrand, Reinhold, New York.

Koenig, H. G. (2001) *Spirituality in Patient Care: Why, How, When and What?* Templeton Foundation Press, Radnor, Pennsylvania.

Legere, T. (1984) A spirituality for today. *Studies in Formative Spirituality,* **5**(3), 375–85.

Leininger, M. (1989) *Qualitative Research Methods in Nursing.* Orlando, Florida.

Macquarrie, J. (1972). *Paths in Spirituality.* SCM, London.

McSherry, W. (1997) *Making Sense of Spirituality in Nursing Practice*. Churchill Livingstone, Edinburgh.

McSherry, W. (2000) *Making Sense of Spirituality in Nursing Practice*. Churchill Livingstone, Edinburgh.

McSherry, W. and Draper, P. (1998) The debates emerging from the literature surrounding the concept of spirituality as applied to nursing. *Journal of Advanced Nursing*, **27**, 683–91.

Millison, M. B. (1988) Spirituality and the caregiver, developing an underutilised facet of care. *The American Journal of Hospice Care*, March/April, 37–44.

Mische, P. (1982) Toward a global spirituality. In *The Whole Earth Papers* (ed. P. Mische). East Grange NJ Global Education Association. No 16.

Montgomery, C. L. (1991) The care-giving relationships: paradoxical and transcendent aspects. *Journal of Transpersonal Psychology*, **23**(2), 91–105.

Morrison, R. (1989) Spiritual health care and the nurse. *Nursing Standard*, **5**, 34–5.

Narayanasamy, A. (1993) Nurses' awareness and preparedness in meeting their patients' spiritual needs. *Nurse Education Today*, **13**, 196–201.

Narayanasamy, A. (1999a) A review of spirituality as applied to nursing. *International Journal of Nursing Studies*, **36**, 117–25.

Narayanasamy, A. (1999b) ASSET: a model for actioning spirituality and spiritual care education and training in nursing. *Nurse Education Today*, **19**, 274–85.

Narayanasamy, A. (2000) The cultural impact of Islam on nursing education. *Nurse Education Today*, **7**, 57–64.

Piles, C. (1986) Spiritual care: role of nursing education and practice: a needs survey for curriculum development. *Unpublished doctoral dissertation*, St Louis University.

Ross, L. (1997) *Nurses' Perceptions of Spiritual Care*. Avebury, Aldershot.

Samarel, N. (1991) *Caring for Life and Death*. Hemisphere Publishing Corporation, New York.

Shelly, J. A. (2000) *Spiritual Care: A Guide for Caregivers*. InterVarsity Press, Illinois.

Shelley, A. L. and Fish, S. (1988) *Spiritual Care: The Nurse's Role*. Inter Varsity Press, Illinois.

Silverman, D. (1933) *Interpreting Qualitative Data*. Sage, London.

Soeken, K. L. and Carson, V. J. (1987) Responding to the spiritual needs of the chronically ill. *Nursing Clinics of North America*, **22**(3), 603–11.

Stoll, R. G. (1979) Guidelines for spiritual assessment. *American Journal of Nursing*, **79**, 1574–7.

Teasdale, K. (1992) Reassurance in nursing. *Unpublished PhD Thesis*. Sheffield Hallam University.

CHAPTER 6

Spirituality and learning disabilities: a qualitative study

Aru Narayanasamy, Bob Gates and John Swinton

Summary

This chapter describes a unique empirical study where critical incidents were obtained from learning disability nurses to understand how they attempt to meet the spiritual needs of the people for whom they care. Following analysis, the nurses' approaches to meeting spiritual needs were categorised as 'personal' or 'procedural', and each of these is described in turn. There then follows a discussion on the effects of these nurses' interventions on both clients and their families, and nurses themselves. The findings of the study illuminate how these learning disability nurses attempted to meet the spiritual needs of people with learning disabilities in their care. The findings may help nurses ensure that spiritual needs are identified in the construction of the personal care plans of people with learning disabilities.

Key points

- Attention to spiritual needs is important to learning disabilities care.
- There is a need for a research-based spiritual care in learning disabilities.
- Spiritual care interventions produce a positive effect on clients and nurses themselves.
- The personal approach arising from this study offers an ideal model for spiritual care.

Introduction

Within the caring professions the notion of holistic health care has gained popularity, and this is especially so in learning disability nursing (Gates and Beacock, 1997). More recently, in a study on the unique role of the learning disability nurse in the multidisciplinary team undertaken by Alaszewski *et al.* (2000), holistic care was identified as the hallmark of this specialty of nursing. Such holism implies care that should embrace attention to body, mind and spirit. Emerging research highlights the importance of spiritual care in nursing and suggests that there is scope for improving this dimension of care in order to improve the quality of life for many clients, including those with learning disabilities (Swinton, 2001a, 2002).

However, there is little evidence in the nursing literature that clearly shows how nurses caring for people with learning disabilities respond to clients' spiritual needs. The purpose of this study was to begin to open up this area of research and explore the ways in which learning disability nurses construct and respond to their clients' spiritual needs.

Literature review

There is a good deal of diversity among the various spiritual traditions and perspectives represented within the literature. There is, however, a general consensus that spirituality is a significant dimension of human wellbeing which is necessary for authentic and genuinely holistic care of body, mind, and spirit (Montgomery, 1991; Koenig, 1997; Narayanasamy, 1999a; McSherry, 2000; MacKinlay, 2001; Swinton, 2001a).

Current nursing literature would seem to equate a state of wellbeing with the harmonious balance between these three interrelated, but nonetheless distinct, entities: body, mind and spirit (Department of Health, 1993; Oldnall, 1996); distress in any one of these areas affects the others. Therefore, a holistic approach designed to restore the harmonious balance between these three components of people is paramount if wellbeing is to be restored.

There is some convergence in the nursing literature that spirituality is an elusive concept, especially when nurse theorists attempt to define it (Oldnall, 1995; McSherry and Draper, 1998; MacKinlay, 2001; Narayanasamy, 2001). This problem is further compounded by the common misperception that the word is necessarily equated with institutional religions such as Christianity and Judaism (Taylor *et al.*, 1995; Swinton, 2001b). Several studies have confirmed confusion among nurses where spirituality is conflated with religion (Harrison

Table 6.1 Definitions of spirituality.

■ The essence or life principle of person (Colliton, 1981)

■ A sacred journey (Mische, 1982)

■ The experience of the radical truth of things (Legere, 1984)

■ Giving meaning and purpose (Legere, 1984)

■ A belief that relates a person to the world (Soeken and Carson, 1987)

■ Being rooted in an awareness that is part of the biological make up of the human species (Narayanasamy, 1999a)

■ That which gives meaning, purpose, hope and value to people's lives. This is part of a wide concept which may include but is not defined by religious faith and culture (Swinton, 2002)

and Burnard, 1993; Narayanasamy, 1993; Ross, 1997). Various definitions of spirituality are given in Table 6.1.

For current purposes, a useful working definition is found in Swinton (1999): spirituality refers to that aspect of human existence that gives it its 'humanness'. It concerns the structures of significance which give meaning and direction to a person's life and helps him or her deal with the vicissitudes of existence. As such it includes vital dimensions such as the quest for meaning, purpose, self-transcending knowledge, meaningful relationships, love and commitment, as well as the sense of the Holy amongst us. A person's spirituality is that part of them which drives them on towards their particular goals, be they temporal or transcendent. This definition will be used to underpin the subsequent discussion.

Spirituality and learning disabilities

There is a significant shortage of literature on spirituality and disability (Selway and Ashman, 1998). When it comes to the area of spirituality in learning disabilities, this lack is even more acute (Swinton, 2001a). This could be because providing for clients' spiritual needs is not perceived as essential (Balkizas and O'Hare, 1994). It may be something to do with the 'anti-tenure effect' as described by Larson *et al.* (1992), i.e. the implicit, unwritten rule that any academic scientist who wants to gain tenure/academic credibility within their institution will not focus on something as 'unscientific', 'immeasurable' and 'ethereal' as spirituality. It may also be that 'some element of embarrassment keeps researchers from probing this area of investigation or perhaps it is the complexity of the topic itself' (Selway and Ashman, 1998). It may also relate to a general unwillingness to address spiritual issues, which is indicative of a wider failure to address emotional needs in people with learning disabilities (Curtice, 2001).

Whatever the reason, the paucity of literature suggests that spirituality may be an underused resource in the lives of people with disabilities in general, and learning disabilities in particular. The literature that does exist indicates that spirituality can be a significant dimension in the lives of many people with learning disabilities (Narayanasamy, 1997; Curtis, 2000; Foster, 2000; McNair and Leguti, 2000; Swinton, 2002).

The evidence suggests that the spirituality of people with learning disabilities can be a valuable source of social and psychological support – particularly (but not necessarily so) if the person is involved with a religious or spiritual community (McNair and Leguti, 2000). It can also be a vital source of meaning making (Swinton, 2001a), friendship (Gaventa, 1993; Swinton, 1999), acceptance, and self-worth (Vanier, 1992, 2000).

Even for the most profoundly impaired people, spirituality can play a significant part in their lives (Bassett *et al.*, 1994). There is some evidence that nurses do make efforts to meet the spiritual needs of clients. However, when it is used, there is evidence to suggest that there is a good deal of diversity in the ways that nurses use it and the approaches they take towards intervention.

In a study of nurses' responses to the spiritual needs of their patients, Narayanasamy and Owen (2001) identified a variety of spiritual care approaches from incidents provided by a sample of participants working in adult, mental health and child care settings. The researchers categorised these responses as personal, procedural, culturalist, or evangelical. They found that nurses who took personal and culturalist approaches were willing to give time and personal attention to patients and engage in all aspects of patient care. However, those who used a procedural approach were less personal and tended to be formal and routine-oriented, although these participants believed that they were meeting their patients' spiritual needs.

The evangelical approach taken by some participants raised ethical questions about its appropriateness in terms of respect for autonomy, although this category of participants expressed that they were also meeting patients' spiritual needs.

A further finding of this study was that participants claimed that patients and their families derived positive effects from spiritual care interventions, and nurses themselves derived satisfaction from the experience of spiritual care. It is, of course, not possible to generalise these findings to learning disabilities nursing, as nurses from this discipline were not included in the study. Nevertheless, this study is indicative of the potential that spirituality has for both carer and patient. As such it is worthy of deeper reflection within a learning disabilities context.

Table 6.2 Reasons why spiritual care is not given attention in nursing.

■ Narrow conceptions of spirituality which equate it with religion, fear of incompetence (Granstrom, 1985)

■ Lack of awareness of nurses' own spirituality (Harrington, 1995)

■ Lack of education with regard to spiritual issues (Oldnall, 1996)

■ Role ambiguity

■ Lack of communication and environmental factors (Ross, 1997; Taylor *et al.*, 1995; Harrison, 1993; Narayanasamy, 1993).

The neglect of the spiritual

While there is evidence to suggest the benefits of spirituality for the lives of people with learning disabilities, it is clear that this potential resource is often omitted from nurses' thinking about care. The current findings of nursing research on spiritual dimensions of nursing have consistently suggested that spiritual care is not given adequate attention in nursing. Some of the reasons for this are given in Table 6.2.

Thus, while spirituality is potentially a useful therapeutic resource, the evidence suggests that in practice it is frequently underused. Emerging research from the area of learning disabilities suggests that care and support workers are not equipped to recognise and respond to the spiritual needs of people with learning disabilities. A study by Swinton (2002) confirmed the potential benefits of spirituality for people with learning disabilities, but highlighted some significant barriers to the provision of spiritual care (Table 6.3).

If this is so, there is a significant gap in the way care is currently being provided and the way carers and support workers are presently being trained and educated.

Table 6.3 Barriers to the provision of spiritual needs.

■ Failure to recognise the significance of spirituality in the lives of people with learning disabilities.

■ Support workers' lack of confidence within this area.

■ Uncertainty amongst care providers regarding personal spiritual and religious beliefs and values.

■ Time constraints.

■ Embarrassment over the apparently non-scientific nature of spirituality.

While some research has been done into how nurses in various contexts deal with spiritual issues, it would appear that little is known about the ways in which learning disability nurses deal with the spiritual dimension of their clients' experiences. Providing evidence of the complexity of the role of the learning disability nurse and the contribution they can make to the wellbeing of people with learning disabilities has always been problematic. When it comes to spiritual issues this difficulty is particularly acute. In order to contribute to the filling of this gap in the learning disability nursing literature, the present study was undertaken to illuminate how these nurses construct their understandings of the spiritual needs and the ways in which they provide spiritual care for the people with whom they work.

Given the importance that the White Paper in England (Department of Health, 2001) places on person-centred planning for people with learning disabilities, it is imperative that we have ways of understanding how we can incorporate the spiritual needs of people into such plans.

Aim of the study

The study aimed to explore how learning disability nurses construct and respond to their clients' spiritual needs.

Methods

This study used a qualitative approach that incorporated the critical incident technique as described by Flanagan (1954), Cormack (1996) and Narayanasamy and Owen (2001). The critical incident technique, as a method of data collection, was popularised by Flanagan (1954), and is particularly useful for collecting data from indirect observation of human behaviour in order to facilitate problem solving (Cormack, 1996). According to Cormack (1996):

An incident relates to any observable human activity that is sufficiently complete in itself to permit inferences to be made.

This method is used in preference to direct observation because of the practical difficulties and constraints often experienced by researchers using observation, particularly in clinical settings (Narayanasamy and Owen, 2001). The added advantage of this method is that it depends on descriptions of actual events, rather than descriptions of things as they should be. It is suggested that it recreates the authenticity of practice, because the technique is largely concerned with the real, rather than the abstract, world, and at the same time it acknowledges the constraints and limitations that we encounter in the world in which we live and work.

An invitation letter about the purpose and nature of the study was sent to 50 nurses working with people with learning disabilities at a variety of settings in the East Midlands region of England. A total of 15 nurses expressed an interest in being interviewed and provided examples of critical incidents relating to their experience of implementing spiritual care. Of these 15 nurses, 10 actually participated in the study. These nurses worked with people with moderate to severe learning disabilities, some of whom were described as having challenging behaviour. All lived in residential community settings.

Data collection

Before the completion of the critical incident interviews, participants were given further information about the purpose of the study and the voluntary nature of participation, and assurances were made that anonymity and confidentiality would be maintained. At the interviews, participants were encouraged to reflect on and write down their responses to the following four topic areas:

■ Describe a nursing situation that demonstrated when and how informants recognised that clients had spiritual needs.
■ Explain how and why informants could identify specific spiritual needs.
■ Describe what informants did to try to help their clients meet their spiritual needs.
■ Describe the effects of their actions on the clients or clients' families, and the reasons why informants concluded that their actions had such effects.

At the interview, as soon as the participant completed the critical incidents, the researcher read them and asked for clarification where points were unclear and added further information that participants offered. Following this, participants were asked to verify that the final version of the completed critical incidents were reflective of their lived experience. This was done to ensure that participants were in a meaningful sense co-researchers in the study, as well as to avoid interpolation of critical incidents by the researcher.

Data analysis

Data obtained from the interviews were then subjected to content analysis as suggested in Narayanasamy and Owen (2001). Data were managed in an objec-

Table 6.4 The process and outcomes of responding to clients' spiritual needs.

How nurses became aware of clients' spiritual needs	The nature of clients' concerns	The nurses' actions	The outcome of nurses' interventions
Religious background	Religious needs	Personal approach, e.g. engagement/ supportive, friendship, love, trusting relationship	Effects on clients and family, e.g feeling happier, deriving a sense of strength and support
Cues such as spiritually/religiously loaded content of conversation	Spiritual needs	Procedural approach, e.g. logical steps, arranging opportunities to attend services	Effects on nurses, e.g. happy that we were of help to client, feeling a sense of achievement, a satisfying experience

tive and systematic way that led to the construction of inferences. In the initial analysis several theoretical categories were identified, and these were then condensed into key themes relating to spiritual care (see Table 6.4).

The categories and themes were then subjected to review by a panel who had particular expertise within the subject area. They then tested the validity of the researchers' analysis.

Findings and discussion

The themes and categories that emerged from the critical incidents data and the subsequent emerging theoretical understanding derived from analysis of the data are described and discussed below.

How do learning disability nurses become aware of the spiritual needs of people with learning disabilities?

The description of this area is drawn exclusively from the participants' discussion of critical incidents in the interviews. Learning disability nurses gave accounts of incidents within which they became aware of their clients' spiritual needs. The initiation of spiritual interventions by nurses seemed to depend on specific cues. The learning disability nurses who participated in this study became aware of clients' spiritual needs when they recognised two primary points:

1. The client's religious background
2. Spiritually/religiously loaded conversation

These two categories acted as strong prompters for these nurses to recognise and respond to their clients' spiritual/religious needs. Both of these categories are described and discussed in turn.

Religious background

Nurses gave accounts of their clients' religious background, suggesting that they had needs within this area of their lives. Clients expressed religious faith and practices which led nurses to be sensitive to these needs:

> A client decided that he wanted to attend a local church on a regular basis. He wanted to go with fellow clients who already attended regularly.... Discussion took place about church services before he started going regularly.
>
> They were Jehovah's Witnesses, and very strict in their observations of their rules. They didn't eat meat, etc. I was aware of this as soon as I entered their house.... picture of Jesus Christ on the wall, and I was offered Barley cup, decaffeinated beverages...

The findings suggest that information about clients' religious background acted as a strong indicator for nurses which led them to initiate action that took into account the significance of their clients' spiritual needs. This background information stimulated the delivery of services that could be described as religious in nature rather than spiritual. This observation is not insignificant.

Spiritually/religiously loaded content of conversation

Further analysis of nurses' accounts suggest that spiritually/religious loaded conversation with clients and their families prompted them, in most instances, to initiate actions to meet their clients' needs. This discourse led to measures in terms of practical action or gestures of sensitivity and consideration of the client's/family's spirituality:

> Unfortunately the client's mother died... It has rekindled her previous loving relationship leading to a deep sense of loss... The client felt pun-

ished by God for not being 'good or bad' and that she had somehow contributed to her mother's untimely death. She expressed potentially suicidal feelings due to her increasing desperation and total loss of meaning and purpose in life.

When a client's conversation was found to have strong spiritual/religious dimensions, these nurses used them as prompters to initiate spiritual care interventions. Nurses who are committed to a client-centred approach often picked up verbal and non-verbal cues, which could be described as spiritual in nature to initiate spiritual care interventions. This suggests that nurses who used such approaches are more responsive to clients' spiritual needs, as opposed to religious needs.

This is consistent with Ross's (1997) findings where she found that nurses who demonstrated a person-centred approach give spiritual care to a deeper level than those who do not. However, there is evidence to suggest that nurses are insufficiently sensitised to spiritual issues, which prevents them from effectively responding to religious and spiritual care. It tends to be people who have explored their own spirituality or who have been exposed to spiritual experiences within their own lives who are most likely to pick up on the spiritual needs of others.

Ross (1997) has identified in her study that nurses who claimed religious affiliation were better than those without such affiliation in identifying clients' spiritual needs. Similarly, Harrington (1995) discovered that uncertainty regarding personal spiritual and religious beliefs and values was a significant barrier for the delivery of spiritual care. As nurses are frequently unaware of their own spirituality and spiritual needs, they are often ill prepared to recognise and care for the spiritual needs of others (Narayanasamay and Owen, 2001). It is very difficult to give what one does not have oneself (Swinton, 2001a). Such a suggestion is consistent with findings from other studies where a relationship between nurses' willingness to be involved in general and spiritual care and their personal belief system has been established (Piles, 1986; Forrest, 1989; Piles, 1990; Samarel, 1991; Narayanasamy and Owen, 2001).

It therefore seems reasonable to infer that nurses' personal belief systems may well influence their recognition of the need for, and participation in, spiritual care.

The nature of clients' needs

With regard to the nature of clients' needs, participants presented incidents which could be distinguished as either specifically religious or more generally spiritual.

Religious needs

Cues from clients about their religious beliefs and practices led nurses to formu-
late care plans which characterised sensitivity and consideration to their clients'
religious needs:

> There was a client who was dying, he had Alzheimer's disease and had
> difficulties in communicating. His spiritual needs were recognised... we
> liaised with his sister and he was visited by the local vicar.... His sister
> was religious so we felt that if he had been able to choose, he would
> probably have wanted to be visited by the vicar before he died.
>
> It was established at the assessment that the client and his mother had
> strong Catholic feelings... enjoyed going to church and enjoyed religious
> programmes on TV.

Clients' expression of religious beliefs and practices led these nurses to become
sensitive to their clients' needs. The symbolic aspects of some clients' lives, such as
religious pictures and artefacts, acted as concrete factors that led to a recognition of
religious needs, and these in turn prompted nurses' attention to meet these needs.

Spiritual needs

The findings indicate that some nurses identified clients' spiritual concerns in
non-religious terms that included

> discussion of feelings, expression of depressive moods, reminiscing
> about the past, agitation, anxiety, sorrow, being punished, hopelessness,
> and a sense of losing meaning and direction.

Extracts from nurses' critical incidents illustrate these factors:

> Although the client didn't say much initially, I felt that he was disap-
> pointed that he was unable to accompany his parents... maybe he felt a
> sense of rejection and felt that life was meaningless without his loved
> ones being with him. He probably felt alienated being in unfamiliar sur-
> roundings. The staff felt that it would be desirable to make him feel at
> home. We tried to involve him in various activities but he continued to be
> unhappy and miserable. It was difficult to get him to open up to us...

This aspect of the finding showed that those who identified clients' spiritual concerns in non-religious terms used a more personal approach (client-

centredness). This willingness to engage at a personal level with clients helped them to identify emotional tensions and turmoil and the nurses made efforts to be involved in giving counselling support to clients to overcome their spiritual distress. This is consistent with Ross's (1997) study in which she found that nurses who had clear views about the meaning of life and wider issues often engaged at a deeper level with clients when providing spiritual care.

Spiritual and religious needs

It appears that nurses are likely to be more attuned to recognising religious needs than they are to recognising more general spiritual needs. In almost all cases sensitivity to religious needs and practices was shown. Although this is a good sign, it may be the case that other spiritual needs, such as the search for meaning and purpose, and a need for love and security could have been overlooked.

Current nursing literature considers these factors to be an important part of clients' spiritual dimension (Narayanasamy, 1999b; Swinton, 2001a,b). There is consensus in the nursing literature that although nurses usually display some knowledge of and ability to identify the concrete aspects of clients' religious needs, e.g. communion and dietary needs (Chadwick, 1973; Narayanasamy, 1993; Ross, 1997), they find it more difficult to recognise spiritual needs which could be described as predominantly psychological in nature (Highfields and Cason, 1983). This would appear to find some support from this research project.

The nurses' actions

The findings suggest that nurses, on identification of patients' spiritual and religious needs, used approaches that could be described as personal and procedural. These are analytical categories constructed from the data, but in reality there were elements of more than one approach in some informants' accounts.

Personal approach

Some informants described spiritual needs in non-religious terms. These spiritual needs related to emotional feelings, thoughts, and expressions of the need to search for meaning and purpose:

The client was enabled to develop meaningful relationships and trust to offer as much care and attention she required... psychological reassurance and compassion... this was given at all times.

Nurses who adopted this approach were personally involved in addressing clients' spiritual needs. They were willing to give time and attention to clients and engage in all aspects of client care:

I suppose we included in our care plan to give him: time and space, build a sense of trust and security, and show him love and compassion as best as we can. And support him with the task of building trusting relationships with staff and other residents. He actually began to trust some members of staff... He began to relate to a particular member of staff... it appeared that finally he was able to find something to do, something that gave him a sense of meaning and purpose, and above all, found someone he could relate to and trust...

This approach to spiritual care could be described as holistic. The relationship with clients tended to be one that prompted feelings of trust and security among clients. Nurses used a counselling approach and supported clients during crisis. The findings of this aspect of the study are consistent with the nursing literature which stresses the importance of a personal approach comprising the elements identified earlier (Montgomery, 1991; Narayanasamy and Owen, 2001).

Montgomery (1991) observes that nurses who allow themselves to be close to clients actually experience, on some level, the patient's healing, or the positive effects of their caring. It would seem that this approach could be considered to be an ideal model for spiritual care.

Procedural approach

The procedural approach tended to address needs that could be described as religious in nature. Clients' expression of religious beliefs and practices were perceived as spiritual needs:

... enabled client to attend regular services and other functions linked to church activities.

... his religious dietary needs were considered carefully and we ensured that these were met...

... we encouraged this client to have the television on Sundays when programmes with hymn singing were on because he used to enjoy hymns...

The procedural approach tended to address needs that could be described as religious in nature. Clients' expressions of religious beliefs and practices are perceived as spiritual needs. Participants who used this approach took logical steps to address clients' religious needs. Although the procedural approach is commendable in addressing the religious needs of clients, these participants appeared to be impersonal in their approach, in that generalised religious routines rather than the particular spirituality of the individual set the tone for care intervention. This type of practice raises a question as to whether spiritual distress displayed in non-religious terms and expressions would receive any spiritual care interventions from certain learning disability nurses.

This suggestion finds some support within the nursing literature, which suggests that the misconception that spiritual needs equate to religious needs may mean that those clients who do not express outward signs of spiritual needs are likely to be ignored (Ross, 1997; McSherry, 2000). Even when recognised, non-religious spiritual needs may be misdiagnosed and treated inappropriately.

There is a real temptation to simply translate a person's spiritual experiences into the narrower, but more familiar, language of psychology or psychiatry. Similarly, such distress may be 'psychologised', i.e. interpreted within the boundaries of an explanatory framework which is more familiar to the nurse than a spiritual paradigm. Doing this enables nurses to hold the experience within a linguistic framework that is both familiar and professionally legitimate (Swinton, 2001a). Within such a framework it is possible to make sense of the person's 'spiritual' experiences without the need to take his or her spirituality seriously. There is evidence to suggest that nurses do engage in such a process of reframing spiritual distress (Oldnall, 1995).

It is clear therefore that nurses need to be aware of, and able to recognise, both types of spiritual need if they are to be effective in providing authentic, person-centred, spiritual care.

The outcome of nurses' interventions

Nurses from this study identified that the outcomes of their spiritual care interventions had therapeutic effects on clients, families, and also on themselves on most occasions.

Positive effect on clients

Following spiritual care interventions, clients appear happier, relaxed and peaceful:

The love, understanding and compassion seemed to have helped the client. We always ensured that he was actively involved in the decision-making process, giving as much choice as possible and to treat the place as his own home.

I am not sure if I have done anything specific, but showing him some understanding for his need to have the time and space to adjust to the sense of separation had helped, I think.... Our action appeared to have helped an unhappy young man to be a lot happier. Somehow, he appeared to be calmer, contented... knowing that he could trust staff and the place, and above all he could do something that gave him what I would call greater meaning and peace as well as a sense of fulfilment...

Effects on family

Further to the recognition of the effects of spiritual care interventions on clients, nurses gave accounts which suggested that such interventions had positive effects on clients' families as well:

His family were delighted to see him much happier and continue to visit...

The family were pleased to have an updated care plan and felt at ease when leaving their daughter in our care.

Spiritual care appears to be something which is recognisably life-enhancing for clients and their families. This general state of wellbeing of clients and families is a product of holistic care, of which spiritual care is an important component of total care.

The findings suggest that, following spiritual care interventions, clients appeared peaceful, relaxed and calm, and grateful. Such states would aid clients' healing and recovery (or peaceful death). Added to this, the learning disability nurses in this study reported that many clients felt comforted and supported as a direct result of spiritual care interventions. Other clients reported that they felt stronger and more able to cope as a direct outcome of spiritual care intervention.

From this it could be surmised that spiritual care interventions may have, directly or indirectly, reduced distress and enabled clients to gather emotional strength to cope with difficulties in their lives. This would be in line with the more general literature on the effects of spiritual interventions (Miller, 1999). It may well be that indicators of spiritual wellbeing could be developed using these descriptors.

Presently, indicators of the spiritual wellbeing of people with learning disabilities based on empirical evidence are not readily available. Such descriptors relating to spiritual wellbeing could be used for the development of spiritual care indicators when evaluation of spiritual care is being considered.

Effects on nurses

Apart from clients and relatives, nurses in this study gave accounts that suggest that they felt that giving attention to clients' spiritual needs and its subsequent effects on clients and families was a satisfying experience:

> My colleagues and I felt quite happy that we were able to help a young man to be happy again. His parents were happy to see their son transformed from a sad to a cheerful person. When they received the drawing their son had done, they were amazed. Their faces lit up and captured it all.... We felt that we had helped a young man settle and find a sense of peace. It is satisfying that we have helped a client spiritually. That's what I think spirituality is about, it is not necessarily dealing with religious things, really.
>
> On reflection, after momentarily doubting my abilities to facilitate spiritual recovery, I did feel a sense of achievement through enabling the client to overcome such adverse circumstances. All members of the care team offered compassion, kindness, gentleness, and understanding...

This statement suggests that nurses' personal involvement in supporting clients with spiritual distress and feeling both competent and confident enough to offer time and attention to clients' spiritual needs is a rewarding experience.

There is probably a strong link between the personal approach to spiritual care and the rewarding experience felt by nurses, although almost all nurses in this study suggested that they derived a positive effect from it. This dimension of the study provides supporting evidence that spiritual care should become an integral and rewarding part of the nurses' role.

It could be speculated that if spiritual care is an active component of the learning disability nurses' role it is most likely to be rewarding and satisfying, contributing to overall improved role satisfaction and increased morale among nurses. The significance of this positive experience should be emphasised in nurse education and training programmes on spiritual care.

Overall this finding adds strength to our earlier claim that spiritual care interventions lead to positive outcomes in clients and relatives. It suggests that this form of practice has further effects on nurses where they equally derive a sense of fulfilment.

Limitations of the study

The study sample was small, and thus limited the number of incidents for analysis. The most that can be claimed is that the study is indicative rather than conclusive. There is a need for wider research within this area.

The authors hope to develop the findings in this initial study, and are currently planning a further study which will include an expanded sample designed to elicit more incidents of spiritual care with people with learning disabilities.

While the incidents and analysis were subjected to review by both participants and external reviewers, there remains a need for caution when generalisation of the study findings is being considered.

Overall, this exploratory study offers scope for further in-depth study of this nature.

Conclusion

This research is the first of its kind in this country in studying spiritual care as described by learning disability nurses caring for people with learning disabilities. Two kinds of approach to spiritual care have emerged from this study, and these were based on the critical incidents derived from nurse informants; they can be described as personal and procedural. Whatever the approaches are, there appears to be a consensus that faith and trust in nurses produces a positive effect on people with learning disabilities and their families. This is consistent with Benson and Stark's (1996) work, where a clear link between positive nurse–client relationships and healing was demonstrated.

Likewise, Montgomery (1991) has suggested that nurses' closeness to patients and willingness to share their experiences had a positive effect and promoted healing. This adds weight to the inseparable and interdependent nature of body, mind and spirit. A harmonious balance between these three elements is paramount for the wellbeing of people with learning disabilities. The findings of this present study suggest that these learning disability nurses derived satisfaction from their role when they implemented spiritual care. In this respect, spiritual care interventions promoted mostly a sense of wellbeing.

Methodologically, this study departs from the conventional interview method. Participants were encouraged to reflect and provide written critical incidents of their experience of spiritual care.

The findings of this present study offer the prospect for developing the personal approach care as a model of spiritual care, and this is in keeping with the White Paper for people with learning disabilities (Department of Health, 2001).

Aspects of this approach should be further developed to produce a model of spiritual care that could be piloted and tested for validation.

Finally, this study has illuminated how learning disability nurses attempted to meet the spiritual needs of people with learning disabilities.

Acknowledgement

This study is the larger part of a project on spiritual care research sponsored by Trinity Care, part of the Southerncross Healthcare Group. We would like to thank the nurses who participated in this study.

This chapter was published as an article in *British Journal of Nursing*, **11**(14), 948–57.

References

Alaszewski, A., Gates, B., Ayer, S., Manthorpe, G. and Motherby, E. (2000) *Education for Diversity and Change: Final Report of the ENB-Funded Project on Educational Preparation for Learning Disability Nursing*. Schools of Community and Health Studies and Nursing, The University of Hull.

Balkizas, D. and O'Hare, M. (1994) Learning disabilities: the helping hand of God. *Nursing Standard*, **9**(9), 46–7.

Bassett, R. L., Perry, K., Repass, R., Silver, E. and Welch, T. (1994) Perceptions of God among persons with mental retardation: a research note. *Journal of Psychology and Theology*, **22**(1), 45–9.

Benson, H. and Stark, M. (1996) *Timeless Healing: Power and Biology of Belief*. Simon & Schuster, London.

Chadwick, R. (1973) Awareness and preparedness of nurses to meet spiritual needs. *Nurses Lamp*, **22**(6), 2–8.

Colliton, M. (1981) The spiritual dimension of nursing. In: *Clinical Nursing* (eds. I. Belland and J. Tassos). Macmillan, London.

Cormack, D. (1996) *The Research Process in Nursing*. Blackwell, Oxford.

Curtice, L. (2001) The social and spiritual inclusion of people with learning disabilities: a liberating challenge? *Contact: Interdisciplinary Journal of Pastoral Studies*, **136**, 17–30.

Curtis, M. (2000) The ghost in the machine. *Learning Disability Practice*, **3**(2), 11–12.

Department of Health (1993) *A Vision for the Future*. NHS Management Executive, London.

Department of Health (2001) *Valuing People: A New Strategy for Learning Disability for the 21st Century*. The Stationery Office, London.

Flanagan, J. C. (1954) The critical incident technique. *Psychological Bulletin*, **51**(4), 327–58.

Forrest, D. (1989) The experience of caring. *Journal of Advanced Nursing*, **14**(14), 815–23.

Foster, M. (2000) High spirits. *Learning Disability Practice*, **2**(4), 16–19.

Gates, B. and Beacock, C. (eds.) (1997) *Dimensions of Learning Disabilities*. Baillière Tindall, London.

Gaventa, B. (1993) Gift and call: recovering the spiritual foundations of friendships. In: *Friendships and Community: Connections Between People With and Without Developmental Disabilities* (ed. A. Noval Amado). Paul Brookes, London.

Granstrom, S. (1985) Spiritual care for oncology patients. *Topics in Clinical Nursing*, **7**(1), 39–45.

Harrington, A. (1995) Spiritual care: what does it mean to registered nurses? *Australian Journal of Advanced Nursing*, **12**(4), 5–14.

Harrison, J. (1993) Spirituality and nursing practice. *Journal of Clinical Nursing*, **2**(4), 211–17.

Harrison, J. and Burnard, P. (1993) *Spirituality and Nursing Practice*. Avebury, Aldershot.

Highfields, M. F. and Cason, C. (1983) Spiritual needs of patients: are they recognized? *Cancer Nursing*, **6**(3), 187–92.

Koenig, H. G. (1997) *Is Religion Good for Your Health? The Effects of Religion on Physical and Mental Health*. Haworth Press, New York.

Larson, D. B., Sherrill, K. A., Lyons, J. S., Craigie, F. C., Thielman, S. B., Greenwood, M. A. and Larson, S. S. (1992) Associations between dimensions of religious commitment and mental health reported in the *American Journal of Mental Health and Archives of General Psychiatry*: 1078–1989. *American Journal of Psychiatry*, **149**(4), 557–9.

Legere, T. (1984) A spirituality for today. *Studies in Formative Spirituality*, **5**(3), 375–85.

MacKinlay, E. (2001) *The Spiritual Dimension of Ageing*. Jessica Kingsley, London.

McNair, J. and Leguti, G. (2000) The local church as an agent of natural supports to individuals with development disabilities. *Issues in Transition*, **2**, 11–16.

McSherry, W. (2000) *Making Sense of Spirituality in Nursing Practice*. Churchill Livingstone, Edinburgh.

McSherry, W. and Draper, P. (1998) The debates emerging from the literature surrounding the concept of spirituality as applied to nursing. *Journal of Advanced Nursing*, **27**(4), 683–91.

Miller, W. R. (ed.) (1999) *Integrating Spirituality into Treatment: Resources for Practitioners*. American Psychological Association, Washington DC.

Mische, P. (1982) Toward a global spirituality. In: *The Whole Earth Papers* (ed. P. Mische). Global Education Association, East Orange, New Jersey.

Montgomery, C. L. (1991) The care-giving relationships: paradoxical and transcendent aspects. *Journal of Transpersonal Psychology*, **23**(2), 91–105.

Narayanasamy, A. (1993) Nurses awareness and preparedness in meeting their patients' spiritual needs. *Nurse Education Today*, **13**(4), 196–201.

Narayanasamy, A. (1997) Spiritual dimensions of learning disability. In *Dimensions of Learning Disabilities* (eds. B. Gates and C. Beacock). Baillière Tindall, London.

Narayanasamy, A. (1999a) A review of spirituality as applied to nursing. *International Journal of Nursing Studies*, **36**(2), 117–25.

Narayanasamy, A. (1999b) ASSET: a model for actioning spirituality and spiritual care education and training in nursing. *Nurse Education Today*, **19**(4), 274–85.

Narayanasamy, A. (2000) The cultural impact of Islam on nursing education. *Nurse Education Today*, **7**(1), 57–64.

Narayanasamy, A. (2001) *Spiritual Care: A Practical Guide for Nurses and Health Care Practitioners*, 2nd edn. Quay, Dinton.

Narayanasamy, A. and Owen, J. (2001) A critical incident study of nurses' responses to the spiritual needs of learning disabilities clients. *Advanced Journal of Nursing*, **33**(4), 446–55.

Oldnall, A. (1995) On the absence of spirituality in nursing theories and models. *Journal of Advanced Nursing*, **21**(3), 417–18.

Oldnall, Andrew (1996) A critical analysis of nursing: meeting the spiritual needs of patients. *Journal of Advanced Nursing*, **23**, 138–44.

Piles, C. (1986) Spiritual care: role of nursing education and practice: a needs survey for curriculum development. *Unpublished doctoral dissertation*, St Louis University.

Piles, C. L. (1990) Providing spiritual care. *Nurse Education*, **15**, 36–41.

Ross, L. (1997) *Nurses' Perceptions of Spiritual Care*. Avebury, Aldershot.

Samarel, N. (1991) *Caring for Life and Death*. Hemisphere Publishing Corporation, New York.

Selway, D. and Ashman, A. F. (1998) Disability, religion and health: a literature review in search of the spiritual dimension of disability. *Disability and Society*, **13**(3), 429–39.

Soeken, K. B. and Carson, Y. J. (1988) Responding to the spiritual needs of the chronically ill? *Nursing Clinics of North America*, **22**(3), 603–11.

Swinton, J. (1999) Reclaiming the soul: a spiritual perspective on forensic nursing. In *Forensic Nursing and the Multidisciplinary Care of the Mentally Disordered Offender* (eds. A. Kettles and D. Robinson). Jesicca Kingsley, London.

Swinton, J. (2001a) *Spirituality in Mental Health Care: Rediscovering a Forgotten Dimension*. Jessica Kingsley, London.

Swinton, J. (2001b) Building a church for strangers. *Journal of Religion, Disability and Health*, **4**(4).

Swinton, J. (2002) *A Space to Listen: Meeting the Spiritual Needs of People with Learning Disabilities*. (2002) The Foundation for People with Learning Disabilities, London.

Taylor, E. J., Amenta, M. and Highfield, M. (1995) Spiritual care practices of oncology nurses. *Oncology Nursing Forum*, **22**(1), 31–9.

Thomson, M. (1998) *The Problem of Mental Deficiency – Eugenics, Democracy and Social Policy in Britain Circa 1870–1959*. Clarendon Press, Oxford.

Vanier, J. (1992) *From Brokenness to Community*. Paulist Press, New York.

Vanier, J. (2000) *Becoming Human*. Darton, Longman and Todd, London.

CHAPTER 7

Transcultural nursing: how do nurses respond to cultural needs?

Summary

The aim of the study was to explore how nurses responded to the cultural needs of their clients. From the transcultural point of view, health care providers must deliver a service that is culturally sensitive and appropriate. However, for a variety of reasons, there is growing concern that the cultural health care needs of minority ethnic groups are not met adequately. This study was done to outline nurses' activity in transcultural care. Empirical data were obtained from a sample of registered nurses ($n = 126$) who were invited to complete questionnaires pertaining to cultural care. As a result of data analysis, the quantitative findings are presented as tables and the qualitative data as categories and themes. The findings suggest that most respondents felt that patients' cultural needs should be given consideration. Cultural aspects of care seem to be a feature of the overall nursing picture within a multicultural context of health care. Many participants claimed that they responded to the cultural needs of patients. Some felt that patients' cultural needs are adequately met; such needs are perceived as religious practices, diets, communication, dying needs, prayer and culture. Furthermore, a significant number of respondents suggested that they would like further education in meeting the cultural needs of their patients. This study offers some insights into transcultural health care practice and, in accordance with the findings, identifies strategies for improving these practices for nursing and nurse education.

Key points

- Nurses' responses to the cultural needs of their patients are revealing.
- Nurses' perception of cultural needs included religious practices, diets, communication, dying needs, prayer and cultural practices.

- Many nurses indicated the need for further education in meeting the cultural needs of their patients.
- Transcultural care models originating from the work of Gerrish and Papadopoulos (1999), Papadopoulos and Lees (2002), and Narayanasamy (2002) offer strategies for improving cultural competence in the UK.
- More research is needed in transcultural health care practice.

Introduction

Britain is regarded as one of the most ethnically diverse countries in Europe (Gerrish *et al.*, 1996; Peberdy, 1997; Le Var, 1998). According to Le Var (1998), it is estimated that about 3 million people in England and Wales (approximately 6% of the population) belong to Black and other minority ethnic groups: Indian (30%), West Indian (18%), Pakistani (17%), Chinese (6%), African (5%), Bangladeshi (4%) and Arab (2%). Thus it is within this culturally diverse society that transcultural health care experts assert that health care providers must deliver a service that is culturally sensitive and appropriate.

However, there is growing concern that the cultural health care needs of minority ethnic groups are not met adequately (Gerrish *et al.*, 1996; Fletcher, 1997; Le Var, 1998; Papadopoulos *et al.*, 1998; Gerrish and Papadopoulos, 1999; Serrant Green, 2001; Narayanasamy, 2002). A fuller commitment to implement transcultural nursing based on research will eradicate the existing anomalies in the health care provision for people from minority ethnic groups.

Transcultural nursing

Transcultural nursing is defined (Leininger, 1997) as:

A formal area of study and practice focused on comparative holistic culture care, health, and illness patterns of people with respect to differences and similarities in their cultural values, beliefs, and lifeways with the goal to provide culturally congruent, competent and compassionate care.

According to Herberg (1989), transcultural nursing is characterised by interventions that are:

... sensitive to the needs of individuals, families and groups who represent diverse cultural population within a society...

Cultural needs

The literature identifies the following as cultural needs: the need for equal access to treatment and care; respect for cultural beliefs and practices, including religious, dietary, personal care needs, and daily routines; communication needs; and cultural safety needs.

The need for equal access to treatment and care

Cultural needs in relation to equal access to treatment and care are paramount in transcultural health care (Gerrish *et al.*, 1996; Polaschek, 1998; Royal College of Nursing, 1998; Gerrish and Papadopoulos, 1999; Henley and Schott, 1999; Narayanasamy, 1999a).

Narayanasamy (1999a) identified that racial discrimination is one of the significant obstacles to treatment and care by minority ethnic groups. The experiences related to racial discrimination, racial harassment and oppression are compelling forces that may contribute to negative perceptions of health service treatment and care by Black and minority ethnic groups (Narayanasamy, 1999a). In an analysis of transcultural health care practices, nurses' ethnocentric attitudes and cultural bias represent strong barriers to health care for Black and ethnic minority groups (Abdullah, 1995), and it is these groups that may also experience stress and psychological trauma (Parfitt, 1988).

Respect for cultural beliefs and practices

Numerous writers have identified the significance of transcultural nursing care needs related to cultural beliefs and practices. Henley and Schott (1999) offer a comprehensive guide for health carers with respect to the cultural and spiritual needs of multi-ethnic patients. Baxter (2000) outlines the importance of respect for cultural and religious identity for mental health clients. Likewise, Chady (2001) identifies strategies for transcultural care practices in the light of the National Service Framework for mental health clients (Department of Health, 1999). In a similar vein, Ayer (1997) offers a broad perspective on issues that affect the life chances and circumstances of people from Black and minority ethnic communities who have learning disabilities. This author provides practical suggestions that will guide leaderships for those who work with people with learning disabilities and their families.

Jukes and O'Shea (1998a) assert that learning disability nurses need to respond to the demands of cultural diversity sensitively from within health care provisions and services. In a second article on the same topic, both authors critically review transcultural models of therapies and counselling for learning disabilities clients (Jukes and O'Shea, 1998b). They conclude that service providers need to work together towards developing a multiculturally sensitive responsive service. They imply that this could be achieved if they work from the client's perspective with a practice framework that enables client empowerment.

However, from the literature there is concern that nurses need to develop knowledge and competence to be effective in meeting needs related to cultural beliefs and practices (Ayer, 1997; Le Var, 1998; Gerrish and Papadapoulos, 1999; Narayanasamy, 2002; Papadopoulos and Lees, 2002).

Communication needs

A sensitive approach to clients' needs is considered to be an important aspect of transcultural care and expression via familiar language, including attention to non-verbal communication (Sherer, 1993; Peberdy, 1997; Royal College of Nursing, 1998; Narayanasamy, 2002). Sherer (1993) claims that language differences cause prolonged treatment as opposed to treatment for English-speaking patients, implying that communication difficulties delay prompt treatment and care. The Royal College of Nursing (1998) advocates that proper translation services should be available for clients who have difficulties in communicating in English.

Cultural safety needs

Polaschek (1998) and Narayanasamy (2002) claim that clients need to derive a sense of cultural safety in the health care environment. This environment needs to engage clients as partners in care where efforts are made to establish respect and rapport, cultural negotiation, and where compromise is conducive for promoting a sense of safety (Narayanasamy, 1999b). There is a consensus that a sense of cultural safety is most likely to promote trust and therapeutic relationships which are vital for interventions designed to meet cultural needs (Narayanasamy, 2002).

Transcultural care practice

The emerging literature on transcultural health care practice in the UK suggests useful strategies for this convention (Le Var, 1998; Gerrish and Papadapoulos, 1999; Chady, 2001; Narayanasamy 2002). Le Var (1998) proposes that strategies for actioning transcultural care practices require initiative; enthusiasm; commitment of individuals and groups; strategic planning; organisation and coordination of services; funding; improved education and training of health care professionals; and in-depth knowledge and understanding of recruitment and research.

Gerrish and Papadopoulos (1999) suggest that transcultural health care practitioners need to develop both cultural-specific and generic cultural competence. These entail the development of knowledge and skills related to a particular ethnic group as well as insights into the beliefs and values that operate within clients' cultures. Such insights are important as beliefs and values influence clients' perceptions of health, illness and bodily functions. On the other hand, generic cultural competence is about knowledge and acquired skills that are applicable in cross-cultural transactions.

Furthermore, Chady (2001) and Narayanasamy (2002) suggest that the ACCESS model offers a framework for implementing transcultural health care. Although the ACCESS model was introduced in mental health care practice, it now has a wider appeal. The acronym ACCESS represents (A)ssessment, (C)ommunication, (C)ultural negotiation and compromise, (E)stablishing respect and rapport, (S)ensitivity, and (S)afety. It is claimed that ACCESS attempts to bring out the moral and ethical imperatives inherent in caring professionals (Narayanasamy, 2002). These include the motivation to be caring, compassionate and beneficial to those in health crises.

However, the literature review so far indicates the gap related to research-based evidence on how nurses meet the cultural needs of patients. Therefore, the aim of the present study is to explore how nurses respond to the cultural needs of patients. It is hoped that the findings of this study will contribute to empirical evidence on transcultural nursing.

Method

In this descriptive study a survey questionnaire was used to obtain data on how nurses responded to the cultural needs of their patients. The questionnaire used had been validated in a previous study (Narayanasamy, 1993), and it comprised closed questions to obtain numerical data and opened-ended questions to elicit qualitative data (see Table 7.1).

Sample

The sample for this study is drawn from registered nurses who attended a post-registration programme at the author's institution (Table 7.2). These nurses

Table 7.1 Cultural care questionnaire.

Question	Choices offered on questionnaire
Do you personally feel that patients' cultural needs should be given consideration when you carried out their nursing assessment?	Yes No
How long has it been since you last recognised a cultural aspect of your patients' needs?	Past week Past month Past 6 months Past year Several years Never
To what degree to you feel that patients' cultural needs are met?	Completely Well met Adequately Poorly met Not met at all
Would you like further education in meeting the cultural needs of patients?	Yes No
Please give an example of a nursing situation in which transcultural care was given (give as many details as you can here)	

were from a region with a multiethnic and cultural population. Questionnaires were distributed to 200 nurses and 126 of them responded (response rate 63%). Participants reflected the multiethnic and cultural characteristics of the population. Of the participants, 9% ($n = 11$) were from a minority ethnic background (African Black, Asians and other Black groups).

Data collection

Data collection was commenced after ethical approval from the local research ethics group. Survey questionnaires with an explanatory letter about the purpose of the research were distributed to nurses who were attending post-registration courses at this institution. They were asked to return completed forms within the specified time limit. As part of ethical consideration, in the letter to the sample all participants were reassured of anonymity (of their identity) and the voluntary

Table 7.2 The sample.

Branch	*n*
Adult nursing	90
Mental health nursing	15
Children's nursing	15
Learning disabilities nursing	6
Total	**126**

nature of their participation. It was assumed that returned questionnaires constituted participants' consent to take part in the study.

Data analysis

The quantitative data were subjected to descriptive statistical analysis and the qualitative data were subjected to content analysis (Silverman, 1993; Cavanagh, 1997). Using both analytical procedures the data from the questionnaires were distilled into meaningful interpretations and these were developed to describe the findings. In particular, the responses to the open-ended questions were subjected to systematic analysis and reviews and the data were distilled into fewer content-related categories. Initially several categories were identified and these were then collapsed into five main themes relating to cultural care. These categories and themes were subjected to peer reviews and inter-rater validation. These measures added to the credibility of the analysis used in this research. Following descriptive statistical analysis of the closed-ended questions the findings were presented as percentages (see results section).

Results

Biographical details

The sample of nurses who participated in this study had experience ranging from 1 year to 32 years of nursing patients from a variety of ethnic and cultural backgrounds. The adult care nurses worked in a variety of specialities which included medical and surgical units, adult intensive care units, trauma units, oncology wards, community nursing, coronary care units and health care of the elderly units. Children's nurses worked in all specialities within paediatric services and mental health nurses worked mainly in acute and continuing care settings. The learning disabilities nurses worked in mainly community care settings. The findings with regard to the various aspects of the questionnaires are given in Table 7.3.

Eighty per cent ($n = 101$) of participants agreed that their patients had cultural needs. According to the participants' perspective, 65% ($n = 82$) said that they had recognised a cultural characteristic of their patients from past week to past month. However, 33% ($n = 42$) claimed that it had been 6 months or longer since they had recognised a cultural need. Twenty per cent ($n = 25$) responded that patients' cultural needs are met and 44% ($n = 55$) indicated that cultural needs were adequately met, whereas 33% ($n = 41$) said that these were poorly met. Eighty-four per cent ($n = 106$) indicated that they would like further education to meet the cultural needs of their patients.

The most frequently cited needs attended to were religious followed by dietary. After these, cultural and dying needs were attended to, and communication needs were considered. Twenty-nine participants omitted responses to this part of the questionnaire.

Table 7.3 Results of responses to questions.

Question	Choices offered on questionnaire	n	%
Do you personally feel that patients' cultural needs should be given consideration when you carried out their nursing assessment?	Yes No	101 25	80 20
How long has it been since you last recognised a cultural aspect of your patients' needs?	Past week Past month Past 6 months Past year Several years Never	36 46 28 5 8 1	29 37 22 4 6 1
To what degree to you feel that patients' cultural needs are met?	Completely Well met Adequately Poorly met Not met at all	6 19 55 39 2	5 15 44 31 2
Would you like further education in meeting the cultural needs of patients?	Yes No	106 20	84 16

Discussion

Nurses' awareness of cultural needs

A significant number of participants (80%; $n = 101$) agreed that their patients had cultural needs (see Table 7.3). However, the overall analysis of the range of data obtained from the questionnaire suggests that the respondents' descriptions of their clients' needs were limited to religious and dietary practices and problems such as language difficulties associated with giving nursing care. Cultural care appears to be synonymous with religious care, e.g. prayer and food prohibited by certain religions. These descriptions reflect some deviations that may originate from transcultural literature which refers to cultural needs, such as consideration of cultural sensitivity, cultural safety, opportunities for equal access to treatment and care, reflexive honesty (re-examination of one's own attitudes) and so forth (Gerrish and Papadopoulos, 1999; Narayanasamy, 2002).

Recognition of cultural needs

As shown in Table 7.3, 65% ($n = 82$) of participants claimed they had recognised a cultural characteristic of their patients from the past week to the past month, and this is encouraging. This result implies that nurses actively practise cultural care. However, a closer examination reveals that cultural needs are interpreted and responded to within a restricted frame of reference, as stated earlier. Also, 33% ($n = 42$) of the respondents mentioned that it was 6 months or longer since they had recognised a cultural feature of their patients' needs.

This means that the cultural dimension of care may not be within these nurses' working agenda. The other explanation may be that these nurses are employed by hospitals with infrequent admissions of minority ethnic patients. However, this is a surprising finding in that respondents were largely from a region which is characteristic of a multicultural society. If transcultural health care is omitted, for whatever reason, then there is much scope for improving this aspect of care.

Cultural needs: are they adequately met?

Overall, a response of 64% ($n = 80$) indicated a positive picture and that cultural needs are adequately met (see Table 7.3). On the face of it, this could be interpreted as encouraging and we can take comfort that nurses are responding to patients' cultural needs and indeed vindicate health care services from the allegation in the literature that transcultural care is inadequate in practice (Health Education Authority, 1994; Royal College of Nursing, 1998).

However, these positive findings need to be cautiously interpreted in the light of nurses' conditions and requirements which tend to be narrow and restrictive (Henley and Schott, 1999; Narayanasamy, 2002). The literature asserts that cultural care is more than responding to the patients' religious, dietary and dying needs, which encompass cultural safety, attention to cultural sensitivity, communication, respect for cultural beliefs, equality of access to treatment and care, and anti-oppressive and discriminatory practices (Dalrymple and Burke, 1995; Polaschek, 1998; Gerrish and Papadopoulos, 1999; Narayanasamy, 2002; Papadopoulos and Lees, 2002).

However, in spite of the divergence of nursing practice of transcultural care from those depicted in the literature, critics can rest assured that at least this feature of care is not totally neglected. Further research is needed to confirm if this practice is widespread, as presently we can only make assumptions in the light of these findings.

Nursing situation when transcultural care was given

Respondents cited cultural needs as given in Table 7.4. Of the 126 nurses who returned the questionnaire, 29 of them left this section incomplete. This may be because of poor recall or because transcultural care is not actively practised for less apparent reasons.

Religious needs

The most frequently cited responses were religious needs ($n = 28$; see Table 7.4). Respondents appear to associate religious needs with cultural needs. These

Table 7.4 How do nurses respond to the cultural needs of patients ($n = 126$)?

Nursing situations	No. of responses*
Religious needs	28 (22%)
Dietary needs	26 (21%)
Culture-specific needs	15 (12%)
Dying needs	14 (11%)
Communication problems	13 (10%)

*Responses to the question: give an example of a nursing situation when transcultural care was given

needs are probably recalled easily because of their symbolic and concrete features:

> Moving a bed in a sideroom so that the patient was facing the correct way for praying

> Periods of fasting

> Patient requested to have her head scarf put back on as soon as she became conscious for religious reasons. This was done...

> ... with emphasis on observation – allowing for a Muslim gentleman to carry out his prayer routine...

> ...Koran placed in incubator/cot. Beads placed on top of incubator...

> A Jehovah's Witness who signed a form requesting not to be given a blood transfusion...

According to the literature, cultural aspects relating to religious needs are permeated with assumptions and stereotypes about certain ethnic minority and diverse religious groups (Henley and Schott, 1999; Narayanasamy, 1999a). Although cultural and religious needs are integral to overall wellbeing, it is important for nurses to be aware that some people may share similar religious beliefs but not necessarily cultural ones. For example, in the UK, some people may share similar religious beliefs and practices but may differ in their cultural beliefs and values (Henley and Schott, 1999).

In the present study participants frequently cited that they responded to patients who were identified as Muslims, Hindus and Jews. However, whether assumptions based on stereotypical images of certain groups prevailed or not, participants gave accounts of what they believed to be examples of incidents in which they attempted to address patients' cultural needs. Furthermore, a significant number mentioned that they had recognised these needs recently.

Dietary needs

The second most frequently cited nursing incidents related to dietary needs (*n* = 26; see Table 7.4):

> Offering appropriate food choice from menu where possible; talking with family, explaining that they can if need be, sort out their own catering arrangements

> Trying to obtain relevant diets for patients who have different religious beliefs...

Offering different types of menus to the patient ensuring the food is of halal type only and reassuring the patient of this

The common example on the ward is trying to provide suitable food to meet different cultural needs...

Although 26 participants responded, the above qualitative data are indicative rather than conclusive that nurses appear to be sensitive to the dietary needs of certain cultural groups. This cultural sensitivity may be reflective of the fact that many institutions make provisions for catering to meet the dietary needs of their patients. Dietary needs appear to be concrete examples that nurses can easily cite as instances of cultural dimensions of care. However, further research is needed to establish if this is widespread before conclusions are drawn.

Attending to culture-specific needs

Fifteen incidents of culturally sensitive care practices were cited when participants were asked to give examples of nursing situations when cultural care was provided (see Table 7.4):

I currently keywork a child of Afro-Caribbean origin. In a day unit of approximately 25 children he is the only Black child. He has problems with self-esteem and personal self-worth, and it has been acknowledged that nursing staff do not have an accurate awareness of his cultural needs and so possibly will find it difficult to address the identified needs. We are attempting to find some educational help to address this need, but it needs to be acknowledged that nursing staff are not aware of cultural needs of clients not of their culture.

... a young Muslim girl, refusing to allow washing.

Maintaining privacy and dignity with an Asian gentleman who did not want any assistance when getting bathed even though his condition required it.

More recently a lady of German origin, fairly open in her ways (not disinhibited) had openly breast fed her baby in front of relatives as well as visitors, not related to her on the unit. We felt that this was inappropriate. She explained to us that it was not a problem to her, but their way...

Although 126 nurses participated, only 15 incidents were outlined about culturally sensitive care (see Table 7.4). This finding in relation to culturally sensitive care is indicative that there is much scope for nurses to become competent in transcultural care.

As seen earlier, Gerrish and Papadopoulos (1999) and, more recently, Papadopoulos and Lees (2002), identified two areas pertinent to cultural competence: culture-generic and cultural-specific. Culture-generic competence is the ability to acquire knowledge and skills that are transferable across ethnic groups, and cultural-specific competence is about possession of knowledge and skills unique to a particular ethnic group. An explanation for this aspect of the findings in the present study could be that nurses are ill-equipped to deal with the more significant aspects of culturally specific needs of their patients.

It is well documented that cultural care demands that nurses become aware of aspects of other people's cultures although it is acknowledged that it is almost impossible to be experts in all cultures, as there are more than 3000 of them (Narayanasamy, 1999b). Transcultural care practices require cultural negotiations and compromise, including an understanding of how patients view and explain their problems (Goode, 1993).

Narayanasamy (2002) offers more specific directions on cultural negotiations and compromise within the ACCESS model:

... the prospect of cultural negotiations facilitates formation of a more complementary relationship between patients and professional carers which ultimately empowers patients as valuable users.

Although it was beyond the participants' conditions, transcultural care may extend to, for example, working in partnership with traditional healers such as folk-health practitioners or herbalists, along with orthodox medical therapists. So what is required here is an integrated approach to care which incorporates orthodox and traditional cultural remedies. However, further research is needed in the area of practice development in terms of therapeutic benefits for such initiatives to be fully realised. In the meantime, transcultural care initiatives with an orientation towards patients' cultural values and care expectations may help. Consequently, care plans derived from the close partnership relationship between nurses and patients are central to transcultural care.

Transcultural care requires that nurses should respect the patient as a unique individual with needs which are influenced by cultural beliefs and values (Narayanasamy, 2002). This will enable patients to maintain their self-respect leading to better self-esteem, which is often at a low ebb during illness. Although the survey questionnaire incorporated an open-ended question on nursing situations related to transcultural care to generate rich qualitative data, the analysis revealed only limited evidence on communications and therapeutic relationships (see Table 7.4). It is likely that more direct questions would have elicited improved responses related to such evidence; however, the researcher avoided asking leading questions to minimise bias.

Furthermore, some guidance on transcultural care is available in the literature (Royal College of Nursing, 1998). Cultural sensitivity is considered to be paramount if transcultural nursing practice is to be effective (Ahuarangi, 1996; Le Var, 1998; Gerrish and Papadopoulos, 1999). The primary concern of transcultural health care is to understand and deliver culturally sensitive care to diverse cultural groups. The care needs of patients should be met through culturally adapted approaches. For nursing interventions to be effective, it is imperative that nurses show sensitivity to all aspects of patients' needs as well as the communication process involving them. Nurse education may have to reinforce this message in the curriculum.

The other important aspect of transcultural care is the issue of cultural safety. Cultural safety can be achieved by creating a caring environment in which cultural adaptation takes place between nurses and patients (Narayanasamy, 2002). Although none of the features of cultural safety emerged in the findings of this study, the literature suggests that patients need to derive a sense of cultural safety (Ahuarangi, 1996; Narayanasamy, 2002). Patients who experience a sense of cultural safety are most likely to have trust in nurses and derive further benefits from the nurse–patient relationship.

Dying needs

Fourteen incidents have shown that nurses were giving culturally sensitive care to dying patients and their families. For example, the following incidents demonstrate such sensitivity:

> A lady had died and I enquired whether they wanted us to do anything specific in preparation for her family seeing her. We were asked not to touch the body at all, which we respected.

> The cultural needs of a Muslim family should be considered in their grieving and last rites when their 3-year-old daughter died one morning.

> ... Dying patients' and relatives' needs, changing of bed position to 'Mecca'

> ... the death of a Sikh in theatre.

Participants appeared to have exercised sensitivity and consideration of patients' culture-specific needs and took practical measures to meet these needs. However commendable these interventions are, it is most likely that caring for the dying and their families brings out the sensitivity in nurses rather than the cultural background of the affected individuals and their families. It also appeared that the religious aspects of the dying patients' needs prompted nurses to take the necessary measures. Most hospitals have routines and procedures in place that are related to the religious orientations of dying patients. Procedure manuals are commonly available as resources to guide nurses about routines to be followed when death occurs in the ward. However, dying patients' religious needs were respected.

Communication

The final emerging theme with respect to nursing incidents of cultural care is communication ($n = 13$; see Table 7.4). Some of the respondents perceived that language difficulties stood in the way of giving good nursing care. The following incidents demonstrate this:

> It became difficult as the patient was unable to speak English and explain that she was not able to wash or be taken to toilet by a man, other than a member of her family.

> We had an Indian man who spoke little English, had perceptual problems due to his condition and also had different cultural requirements. We involved translators, liaison nurse, catering manager and staff from chaplaincy department.

> Patient not being able to speak English who needed an interpreter.

> I needed to arrange interpreter services for a patient attending for preoperative assessment who was unable to understand English.

According to the literature, the crux of transcultural care is communication, comprising strategies such as consideration of appropriate body stances and proximities, gestures, languages, listening styles and eye contact (Peberdy, 1997; Narayanasamy, 2002). Participants were not forthcoming with concrete examples of interpersonal transactions between nurses and patients within a transcultural context. However, there were examples where interpreters were used to overcome the communication difficulties experienced by some non-English speaking patients.

It is important for nurses to be aware that groups vary widely in their ideas about appropriate body stances and proximities, gestures, languages, listening styles and eye contact (Sherer, 1993; Narayanasamy, 2002). Language differences prolong treatment: more for some minority ethnic patients than for English-speaking patients undergoing treatment (Sherer, 1993). According to Narayanasamy (2002), this happens:

> ... because health professionals are unable to determine treatment needs in time and initiate further treatment because of patients' language difficulties.

The implications of this are that communication difficulties may actually impede the early detection of health needs, treatment and care.

Where an interpreter is required, it may sometimes seem convenient to use a member of the patient's family as an interpreter to facilitate the communication process. However, the patient may fabricate a new problem to save embarrassment in the presence of a family member. Also, the interpreter may interpret rather than translate a patient's problems (Narayanasamy, 2002). The nurse who is unfamiliar with the language may not realise whose views are being expressed. For this reason, the Royal College of Nursing (1998) advises against the use of informal interpreters and suggests that substantial professional interpreting should be provided.

Further education in cultural dimensions of care

There is encouraging evidence in this study that a significant number of participants (84%; $n = 106$) have the motivation to request courses in transcultural health care (see Table 7.4). Gerrish et al. (1996), Le Var (1998) and Gerrish and Papadopoulos (1999) identify the limitations of nurse education with respect to cultural awareness programmes and recommend a model for transcultural health care practice and education. This model incorporates the development of cultural sensitivity, cultural awareness, re-examination of ethnicity, intercultural communication and measures to eradicate racism, sharpening up of policies to improve procedures related to recruitment, and selection of candidates for pre-registration nursing courses from minority ethnic communities. With more courses and learning material in this subject, nurses can be helped to become more confident and competent in transcultural health care (Gerrish and Papadopoulos, 1999).

Limitations

The limitation of this study is that it is based on a sample drawn largely from adult nursing and the remaining small numbers were from mental health, learning disabilities and children's nursing. Branch-specific studies involving a variety of methods, such as questionnaires, interviews and observations, might have provided a more comprehensive perspective of transcultural care as practised by nurses. The use of multimethods may have provided method triangulation to increase the study's validity and reliability of data sources. The relationship between nurses' experience and education could have been explored to establish the link between attitudes shaped by education and transcultural care practice. Therefore some caution is needed when making generalisations of the findings.

Implications of findings

The general findings of this study suggest that participants' recognition of and responses to the cultural needs of their patients (with regard to diets, religions and dying), appear to be satisfactory in terms of positive responses. Participants gave a true account of their lived experience of what they believed to be transcultural care. However, the study had reservations about these findings in that such accounts may be based on stereotypical assumptions about patients' ethnicity and religions. The incidents cited by nurses about dying needs may have been prompted by altruistic reactions to the dying and their families rather than cultural concerns. Also, in the care of the dying, patients' religious orientation may have been the prompting factor rather than culture.

Some of the respondents appeared to have used the interpreting services to help them communicate with non-English patients when language barriers were encountered. This is commendable, as a number of participants gave accounts of incidents of language barriers that acted as obstacles to good nursing practice. Anti-racists may take the view that such discourse reflects features of racism and intolerance for people who do not share a common language. This poses many challenges with regard to transcultural care. However, an alternative explanation may be that limited services are offered by the interpreting agencies. It is not uncommon for nurses in general to have limited awareness of interpreting services as some may operate as fringe agencies (Narayanasamy, 2000).

Furthermore, some of the languages spoken by Asian patients may not be covered by the interpreting services. Some considerable delay may be encountered when time is spent to seek appropriate interpreters. Respondents' accounts with respect to this finding did not reveal how they used communication skills such as non-verbal cues to facilitate some understanding and consideration. This calls for a re-examination of the use of communication skills as well as the need for raising some awareness of common languages spoken by Asian patients. There may be a need to review the level and availability of interpreting services, and deficiencies remedied by properly funded and structured utilities.

The findings of this study have implications for nurse education in that participants have expressed a need for further professional development. There is scope for an acceleration of course developments within pre- and postregistration nurse education in cultural knowledge awareness and competence as suggested in the literature (Royal College of Nursing, 1998; Gerrish and Papadopoulos, 1999; Papadapoulos and Lees, 2002). This includes cultural safety, communications, cultural awareness, building trusting relationships, rapport and antidiscriminatory practices.

Conclusion

This empirical study offers some insights into accounts of nurse participants' lived experiences and beliefs about transcultural health care. Although these nurses operated from narrow conditions related to transcultural health care, we may take comfort in the fact that at least some aspects of cultural need are handled with consideration and sensitivity. However, this study also points out that there is scope for improving nurses' knowledge and competence in transcultural health care practice. There is encouraging evidence to suggest that nurses who participated in this study have the motivation to seek further courses and guidance in order to become competent in transcultural care.

Finally, further studies, e.g. branch-specific research in mental health, learning disabilities and paediatric nursing, using a variety of methods, are suggested. It is hoped that this study will prompt further research in transcultural health care practice.

Acknowledgements

This study is the larger part of a project on spiritual and cultural care research sponsored by Trinity Care, part of the Southern Cross Healthcare Group. My thanks are extended to all participants in the study and external and internal reviewers for their valuable comments.

This chapter was published as an article in *British Journal of Nursing*, **12**(3), 185–94.

References

Abdullah, S. N. (1995) Towards an individualized client's care: implications for education. The transcultural approach. *Journal of Advanced Nursing*, **22**(4), 715–20.

Ahuarangi, K. C. (1996) Creating a safe cultural space. *Kai Tiaki Nursing New Zealand*, November, 13–15.

Ayer, S. (1997) Cultural diversity: issues of race and ethnicity in learning disability. In: *Dimensions of Learning Disability* (B. Gates and C. Beacock), pp. 181–202. Baillière Tindall, London.

Baxter, C. (2000) Anti-racist practice: achieving competency and maintaining professional standards. In: *Lyttle's Mental Health and Disorder* (eds. T. Thompson and P. Mathias), pp. 350–8. Baillière Tindall, Edinburgh.

Cavanagh, S. (1997) Content analysis: concepts, methods and applications. *Nursing Research*, **4**(3), 5–15.

Chady, S. (2001) The NSF for mental health from a transcultural perspective. *British Journal of Nursing*, **10**(15), 984–90.

Dalrymple, J. and Burke, B. (1995) *Anti-oppressive Practice: Social Care and Law*. Open University Press, Buckingham.

Department of Health (1999) *Modern Standards and Service Models: National Service Framework for Mental Health*. Department of Health, London.

Fletcher, M. (1997) Ethnicity: equal health services for all. *Journal of Community Nursing*, **11**(7), 20–4.

Gerrish, K. and Papadopoulos, I. (1999) Transcultural competence: the challenge for nurse education. *British Journal of Nursing*, **8**(21), 1453–7.

Gerrish, K., Husband, C. and Mackenzie, J. (1996) *Nursing for a Multiethnic Society*. Open University Press, Buckingham.

Goode, E. E. (1993) The cultures of illness. *US News World Report*, **114**, 74–6.

Health Education Authority (1994) *Black and Ethnic Minority Groups in England*. Health Education Authority, London.

Henley, A. and Schott, J. (1999) *Culture, Religion and Patient Care in a Multiethnic Society*. Age Concern, London.

Herberg, P. (1989) Theoretical foundations of transcultural nursing. In: *Transcultural Concepts in Nursing Care* (eds. J. S. Boyle and M. M. Andrews), pp. 3–53. Scott, Foresman/Little, Brown College Division, Illinois.

Jukes, M. and O'Shea, K. (1998a) Transcultural therapy 1: mental health and learning disabilities. *British Journal of Nursing*, **7**(11), 901–6.

Jukes, M. and O'Shea, K. (1998b) Transcultural therapy 2: mental health and learning disabilities. *British Journal of Nursing*, **7**(20), 1268–72.

Leininger, M. (1997a) Transcultural nursing research to nursing education and practice: 40 years. *Image Journal of Nursing Scholarship*, **29**(4), 341–7.

Le Var, R. M. H. (1998) Improving educational preparation for transcultural health care. *Nursing Education Today*, **18**, 519–33.

Narayanasamy, A. (1993) Nurses' awareness and educational preparation in meeting their patients' spiritual needs. *Nursing Education Today*, **13**, 196–201.

Narayanasamy, A. (1999a) Transcultural mental health nursing 1: benefits and limitations. *British Journal of Nursing*, **8**(11), 664–8.

Narayanasamy, A. (1999b) Transcultural mental health nursing 2: race, ethnicity and culture. *British Journal of Nursing*, **8**(12), 741–4.

Narayanasamy, A. (2000) Cultural impact of Islam on the future directions of nurse education. *Nursing Education Today*, **20**, 57–64.

Narayanasamy, A. (2002) The ACCESS model: a transcultural nursing practice framework. *British Journal of Nursing*, **11**(9), 643–50.

Papadopoulos, I. and Lees, I. (2002) Developing culturally competent research. *Journal of Advanced Nursing*, **37**(3), 258–63.

Papadopoulos, I., Tilki, M. and Taylor, G. (1998) *Transcultural Care: A Guide for Healthcare Professionals*. Quay, Wiltshire.

Parfitt, A. (1988) Cultural assessment in the intensive care unit. *Intensive Care Nursing*, **4**, 124–7.

Peberdy, A. (1997) Communicating across cultural boundaries. In: *Debates and Dilemmas in Promoting Health: A Reader* (eds. M. Siddle, L. Jones, J. Katz and A. Peberdy), pp. 99–107. Open University, Buckinghamshire.

Polaschek, N. R. (1998) Cultural safety: a new concept in nursing people of different ethnicities. *Journal of Advanced Nursing*, **27**(3), 452–7.

Royal College of Nursing (1998) *The Nursing Care of Older People from Black and Minority Ethnic Communities*. Royal College of Nursing, London.

Serrant Green, L. (2001) Transcultural nursing education: a view from within. *Nursing Education Today*, **21**(8), 670–8.

Sherer, J. L. (1993) Crossing cultures: hospitals begin breaking down the barriers to care. *Hospitals*, **67**(10), 29–31.

Silverman, D. (1993) *Interpreting Qualitative Data*. Sage, London.

CHAPTER 8

The **ACCESS** model: a transcultural nursing practice framework

Summary

As transcultural nursing is beginning to be a feature of health care in multiethnic and multicultural Britain, the need for transcultural health practice models is increasing. The focus of this article, the ACCESS model (Narayanasamy, 1999), was developed to offer nurses a framework to deliver transcultural nursing care. Since its introduction there has been increasing interest about it from practitioners, nurse educators and students of nursing. The aim of this study was to ascertain the usefulness of the ACCESS model by a questionnaire study. In the institution where this study took place, pre- and post-registration nursing students are introduced to this model along with other models of transcultural health care. Participants (n = 166) who received transcultural health care education completed questionnaires with statements about the usefulness of this model. A significant number of participants found the model to be very useful with respect to its various features. The conclusion of this study is that the ACCESS model offers a useful framework for nurses implementing transcultural care practice. It appears that students and practitioners are interested in this model because of its practice implications.

Key points

■ Transcultural health care must be given more emphasis in multiethnic and multicultural Britain.

■ There is a need for a culturally sensitive approach to the care of minority ethnic patients based on equality of opportunities with regard to accessing health services, treatment and care.

■ The ACCESS model is about assessment, communication, cultural negotiation and compromise, establishing respect and rapport, sensitivity and safety.

■ The ACCESS model offers a useful framework for nurses implementing transcultural care practice.

Introduction

Britain is regarded as a multi-ethnic and multicultural society with about 3 million people (6% of the population) belonging to Black and other minority ethnic groups (Le Var, 1998). These figures are based on the 1991 census; however, new figures are imminent following the results of the 2001 population census. It is clear that within this society, health care providers need not only to respond to cultural and ethnic diversity but also to deliver a culturally appropriate and sensitive service based on fairness and justice.

Transcultural nursing has been an essential activity within the global context in the 21st century because of various factors. Leininger (1997) outlines such factors as:

■ The marked mobility of people worldwide

■ The increase of migrants, refugees, and displaced people worldwide

■ The need for recognition and respect for cultural identities in terms of values, beliefs and lifeways

■ The changing roles of women and men

■ The increased use of high technology, electronic communication and rapid transportation

■ The growing evidence of cultural conflicts, racism and backlash in human services, but especially in health care

■ The increased demand of health personnel to view clients beyond the traditional 'mind–body medical' perspectives to that of an holistic, multifactor, transcultural care view.

According to the literature (Leininger, 1997), this could be achieved by transcultural nursing. Transcultural nursing is defined by Leininger as:

A formal area of study and practice focused on comparative holistic culture, care, health, and illness patterns of people with respect to differences and similarities in their cultural values, beliefs, and lifeways with the goal to provide culturally congruent, competent, and compassionate care.

Transcultural nursing can be conceptualised as a strategy of caring which takes into account, with sensitivity and consideration, the individual's culture, specific values, beliefs and practices. It is holistic in nature to embrace a comprehensive range of cultural factors, as well as spirituality, economics, politics and kinship in diverse contexts. Transcultural nursing is based on the philosophical, theoretical and empirical perspectives of Leininger (1997) and others in this field. In essence, it offers a strategy to capture people's emic (insider) and etic (outsider) views to plan and implement cultural sensitive care that is congruent to the cultural beliefs and values of clients and their families.

However, there is a consensus of opinions that the provisions for transcultural nursing care are far from satisfactory for a variety of factors in the UK (Gerrish *et al.*, 1996; Le Var, 1998; Gerrish and Papadopoulos, 1999; Chady, 2001; Serrant Green, 2001). Transcultural nursing as a perspective is yet to be widely established, although various bodies stress its importance (UKCC, 1999; English National Board, 2000).

Inadequate educational, research and practice provisions have been blamed in the past for the slow phase in the development of transcultural nursing. However, a small body of evidence with respect to transcultural nursing is emerging in the UK. Most notably, the work of Gerrish and Papadopoulos (1999), Le Var (1998) and McGee (1993, 2000) is beginning to influence education and practice. There are also encouraging signs of practice development with regard to transcultural nursing, one of which is the Cultural Competency and Awareness Project (CCAP) at the Middlesex University Research Centre for Transcultural Studies in Health (Papadopoulos and Lees, 2002). The Royal College of Nursing is continuing to announce in its fortnightly bulletin that it is promoting regional supportive forums with opportunities for nurses to initiate culturally sensitive care.

Antiracist writers claim that racism in society and health care is one of the barriers to the provision of transcultural health care (Ahmad, 1993; Fernando, 1995; Baxter, 2000; Bhopal, 2001). Both personal and institutional racism are blamed for the poor provision (Beishon *et al.*, 1995). Fernando (1995) argues that the starting point in the provision of transcultural care is to recognise racism at its roots as a major cause of discrimination against black and other minority ethnic people. Bhopal (2001) draws attention to racism in medicine and calls for radical measures to exorcise this spectre from health care.

Other focused studies suggest that nurses and health carers are unable to deliver full transcultural care because of a lack of cultural awareness knowledge and competence and poor educational preparation (Gerrish *et al.*, 1996; Papadopoulos *et al.*, 1998; Gerrish and Papadopoulos, 1999). Evidence is emerging that nurses need a practical model of transcultural care practice to guide them to meet the cultural needs of their patients.

It appears that, generally, nurse education and training for nurses are rather patchy and unsystematic, which prevents nurses being effective in transcultural health care practice (Gerrish, 1997). However, some models of transcultural health care exist. The Sunrise Model, as proposed by Leininger (1995), is comprehensive and offers a conceptual framework to guide nurses with regard to transcultural care. Gerrish and Papadopoulos (1999) and Le Var (1998) offer theoretical models based on practice and education to guide nurses in this area of care. In particular, Gerrish (1997) offers a range of teaching and learning strategies for transcultural health care education and training in the evidence.

The PTL model (Middlesex University, 2001; Papadopoulos and Lees, 2002) offers opportunities for nurses to develop cultural competence and awareness with regard to health care. However, these are taking time to influence health care practice with regard to transcultural care. Furthermore, there is a perception that some of these models are too abstract or complicated and nurses find them to be inappropriate or complex to put into practice.

The ACCESS model, originating from the work of Narayanasamy (1999), is considered to be useful because it is practical. The relevance and importance of this model is being acknowledged in the emerging literature on transcultural care (Gerrish and Papadopoulos, 1999; Stanley, 2000; Chady, 2001; Serrant Green, 2001). The current transcultural health education in our institution is based on the ACCESS model (Table 8.1). It is action-centred to facilitate the planning and implementation of culturally congruent care that is sensitive and compassionate in nature.

Table 8.1 The ACCESS model of transcultural nursing (Narayanasamy, 1999).

Assessment:	Focus on cultural aspects of clients' lifestyle, health beliefs and health practices.
Communication:	Be aware of variations in verbal and non-verbal responses.
Cultural negotiation and compromise:	Become more aware of aspects of other people's culture as well as understanding of clients' views, and explain their problems.
Establishing respect and rapport:	A therapeutic relation which portrays genuine respect for clients' cultural beliefs and values is required.
Sensitivity:	Deliver diverse culturally sensitive care to culturally diverse groups.
Safety:	Enable clients to derive a sense of cultural safety.

The ACCESS model

The ACCESS model is represented in Table 8.1. The components of the model are briefly discussed below.

Assessment

A comprehensive assessment of the cultural aspects of a patient's lifestyle, health beliefs and health practices will go a long way in enabling nurses to make decisions and judgments related to care interventions. Cultural assessment may enhance nurses' understanding of the patient's health beliefs and practices. For example, as well as questions about patients' lifestyles, the questions listed in Table 8.2 may be asked for a patient who has diabetes.

An assessment incorporating the questions in Table 8.2, with regard to the patient's beliefs about diabetes and its causes, symptoms and treatment, may be thought of as the patient's explanatory model of illness (Kleinman *et al.*, 1978). The term 'explanatory model' is preferable to the term 'folk' health beliefs as the latter has derogatory connotations relating to something primitive and non-scientific. The information obtained from assessment will provide vital understanding of similarities and differences between the patient's beliefs and attitudes regarding the illness and the nurse's own beliefs and attitudes.

The ACCESS model offers opportunities for a conscious and sustained effort on the part of the nurse to focus on the cultural factors that influence a

Table 8.2 Questions about a patient's health beliefs.

1.	What do you think caused your diabetes?
2.	Why do you think it happened when it did?
3.	What effects will having diabetes have on you?
4.	What kind of treatment do you think you should receive?
5.	Do you believe diabetes can be serious? Why?
6.	Do you think your illness will last over a long period of time?
7.	What are some of the problems that your illness has caused?
8.	Some people forget to take daily medications/injections; does this happen to you?
9.	What have you done to help you remember to take your pills?
10.	What things about diabetes that frighten or worry you?

patient's behaviour and reaction to an illness. Patients' narratives about the progress and difficulties they experience on a daily basis may provide clues about basic values and attitudes regarding the impact of their illness on activities and daily living. The resulting care plans and interventions from this assessment should be considered in the light of the subsequent elements of the ACCESS model.

Communication

The crux of transcultural care is communication (Sherer, 1993; Peberdy, 1997). It is important for nurses to be aware that groups vary widely in their ideas about appropriate body stances and proximities, gestures, language, listening styles, and eye contact. For example, traditional Asians typically consider direct eye contact inappropriate and disrespectful.

It is well known that language differences cause prolonged treatment as opposed to treatment for English-speaking patients (Sherer, 1993); in other words, this happens because health professionals are unable to determine treatment needs in time and initiate treatment because of patients' language difficulties. Sometimes it may seem convenient to use a member of the patient's family as an interpreter to facilitate the communication process; however, in order to save embarrassment in the presence of a family member the patient may fabricate a new problem. Also, the interpreter may interpret rather than translate the patient's problems. The nurse who is unfamiliar with the language may not realise whose views are being expressed.

Cultural negotiation and compromise

This requires that nurses make efforts to become more aware of aspects of other cultures, although it is recognised that it is almost impossible for all of us to be experts in all cultures.

Transcultural therapeutic interventions need cultural negotiation and compromise (Goode, 1993). This requires an understanding of how the patient views and explains the problem. It may include, for example, working in partnership with traditional healers and other health practitioners or herbal therapists along with orthodox medical treatment. It may also involve helping patients to arrange for culturally oriented ceremonies connected with grieving and loss. Nursing intervention should, therefore, be aimed at being oriented to patients' value positions, showing sensitivity to the communication process and care expectations.

Establishing respect and rapport

Disrespect evokes feelings of being devalued, leading to dents in self-esteem. On the other hand, being respected produces a more positive effect. Nurses can portray a genuine respect for the patient as a unique individual with needs that are influenced by cultural beliefs and values (Narayanasamy, 1999). This will enable clients to maintain their self-respect, leading to better self-esteem, which is often at a low ebb during a health crisis. A positive nurse–patient relationship is most likely to establish the rapport between them. This, in turn, will foster an atmosphere of trust in which a therapeutic relationship will be continued. All of these will lead to the development of mutual respect for each other's cultural beliefs and values.

Sensitivity

The primary concern of health care is to understand and deliver diverse culturally sensitive care to diverse cultural groups. The care needs of the patients should be met through culturally adapted approaches. For nursing interventions to be effective, it is paramount that nurses show sensitivity to all aspects of patients' needs as well as the communication process involved. As part of this process, nurses require knowledge of expected patient-specific patterns of communication. For example, it is important for nurses to recognise that certain terms, concepts and distinctions drawn in other languages are not always easily translated into English. In such situations, patients whose first language is not English may sometimes draw from their indigenous vocabulary to make their points. Further understanding of the ways in which style and tone of communication may be used is required.

Safety

Patients need to derive a sense of cultural safety. Conceptualisation related to this part of the model is derived from the work of Ramsden (1993) and Polaschek (1998). Cultural safety as a concept was developed by Moari nurses in an attempt to bring focus to the needs of the indigenous minority in New Zealand. Its strategy is to avert actions that diminish, demean or disempower the cultural identity and wellbeing of an individual. Therefore, culturally safe nursing practice promotes actions which recognise, respect and nurture the unique cultural identity of individuals, and 'safely meet their expectations and rights' (Polaschek, 1998).

It is culturally unsafe if individuals perceive the health care environment as alien and one that ignores their needs in terms of service, treatment or attitude. On the other hand, an environment in which cultural adaptation takes place between nurses and patients may promote a sense of cultural safety. Patients who experience a sense of cultural safety are most likely to have trust in nurses and derive further benefits from the therapeutic relationship which is vital for interventions designed to meet cultural needs.

However, the criticism of this model is that it is not overt about the effects of racism and discrimination with regard to the care and treatment of minority ethnic groups. There could be the emphasis in the model about strategies for equal access to fair and just treatment and care in health care practice for users from black and minority ethnic communities. It needs to be explicit that all forms of obstacles and barriers, including racial discrimination, should be removed to promote equal access to services and practices.

Study methods

This study was carried out as part of an action research into cultural care. Action research is situational in that it is concerned with identification of a problem related to a specific context and instituting measures to solve it in that context (Cohen and Manion, 1989; Rolfe *et al.*, 2001). Action research uses a collaborative and participatory process in which researchers and participants work together by actioning, evaluating and modifying practices continuously to bring about changes (Altrichter *et al.*, 1993; Rolfe *et al.*, 2001; Waterman *et al.*, 2001). The present study uses the following processes of action research:

- Evaluating action in terms of its usefulness (data collection)
- Analysis of data
- Interpretation
- Action (practice education)
- Evaluation (further research).

Data collection

In order to ascertain the usefulness of the ACCESS model a questionnaire study was carried out. The questionnaire used had been piloted and validated in a previous study (Narayanasamy, 1998, 1999). Both third-year students ($n = 69$) and registered nurses ($n = 97$) who had participated in the pre- and post-registration

Table 8.3 Sample.

Sample	Number
Registered Nurses	97
Student nurses (3rd year)	69
Total	**166**

Table 8.4 Questionnaire statements.

1. Developing the cultural aspects of client's life style, health beliefs and health practices.
2. Developing an awareness of variations in verbal and non-verbal responses.
3. Developing awareness of aspects of other people's culture as well as understanding of clients view and explaining their problems.
4. Forming a therapeutic relationship which portrays genuine respect for the client's cultural beliefs and values.
5. Delivering diverse culturally sensitive care to culturally diverse groups.
6. Fostering a culturally safe environment.

transcultural nursing education programme based on the ACCESS model were asked to complete a questionnaire at the end of the programme (Table 8.3).

An explanatory note accompanied the questionnaire with information about the purpose of the study, the voluntary nature of participation, respondents' anonymity and confidentiality. The questionnaire comprised statements as set out in Table 8.4. Participants were asked to indicate in the questionnaire how useful each of the items in the ACCESS model was to them on a scale of 1–5 (1 = no help; 5 = a lot of help). Participants were then asked to return the questionnaire in a stamped addressed envelope to the research team.

Data analysis

Data obtained from the questionnaires were subjected to descriptive statistical analysis in terms of number counts related to the responses to statements about the usefulness of the various components of the ACCESS model. Statistical analysis ensured that the data were presented in an objective and systematic manner. The resulting data were interpreted and presented in graphical formats.

Two internal reviewers with expertise in transcultural health care and action research were invited to check the data analysis and interpretations. Following modifications in terms of reviewers' comments the report of the findings was finalised for dissemination.

Results and discussion

The findings from Figure 8.1 suggest that both qualified nurses and student nurses found the assessment component of the ACCESS model useful or highly useful (90%; $n = 149$). This aspect of the findings indicates that course participants agree that the focus on clients' lifestyles, health beliefs and health practices is valuable.

There is a consensus in the theoretical and practice literature that a comprehensive assessment of patients' cultural factors related to all aspects of their lives is needed. This will go a long way in enabling health care practitioners to make decisions and judgments that would impact upon their care in beneficial ways. Therefore the findings with regard to this aspect of the model strengthen the case for a comprehensive cultural assessment of patients.

A majority of registered nurses (76%; $n = 74$) and student nurses (74%; $n=51$) (Figure 8.2) indicated that the model's emphasis on an increasing aware-

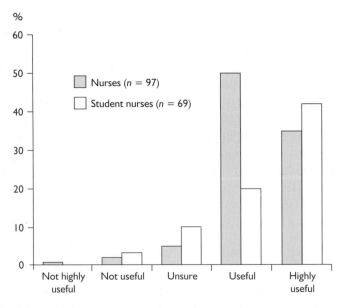

Figure 8.1 Assessing cultural aspects of client's lifestyle, health beliefs and health problems.

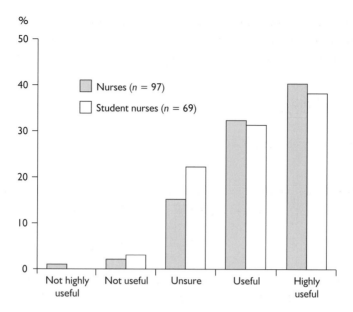

Figure 8.2 Developing an awareness of variations in verbal and non-verbal responses.

ness of variations in verbal and non-verbal responses is useful or highly useful. According to Peberdy (1997) and Sherer (1993), the crux of transcultural care is communication. Furthermore, the Royal College of Nursing (RCN, 1998) has developed a resource guide to aid nurses to use effective communication techniques in caring for patients from multiethnic backgrounds. The present study confirms the importance of cross-cultural communication and the ACCESS model offers the rudiments of communication skills for nurses to engage in transcultural care.

The findings regarding cultural negotiations and compromise (Figure 8.3) suggest that a significant number of participants found this component of the ACCESS model useful or highly useful. Ahuarangi (1996), Gerrish *et al.* (1996) and Gerrish and Papadopoulos (1999) stress that transcultural therapeutic interventions require cultural negotiations and compromise. The prospect of cultural negotiations facilitates the formation of a more complementary relationship between patients and professional carers which ultimately empowers patients as valuable users. According to Polaschek (1998), cultural care with regard to cultural safety is about power relationships in nursing service delivery where the less powerful genuinely have their voices heard about health care and its environment.

It can be inferred from the findings in Figure 8.4 that this aspect of transcultural care would enhance nurses' role in therapeutic interventions in the care of minority ethnic patients when using the ACCESS model. There is consensus in

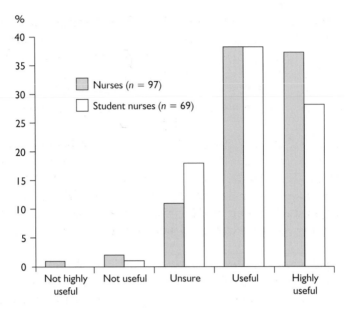

Figure 8.3 Developing awareness of aspects of other people's cultures as well as understanding of clients' views of explaining their problem.

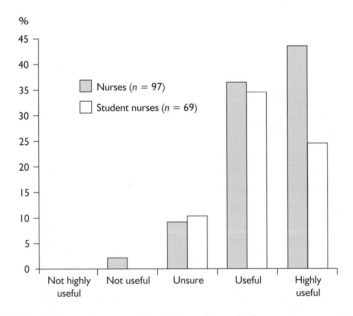

Figure 8.4 Forming a therapeutic relationship which portrays genuine respect for clients' beliefs and values.

the literature (Gerrish *et al.*, 1996; Polaschek, 1998; Narayanasamy, 1999) that in order to establish rapport in therapeutic relationships, nurses must portray a genuine respect for their patients. The ACCESS model focuses on this aspect of care and indicates that respect can be established by treating patients as individuals with needs which are influenced by cultural beliefs and values. The model enables nurses to be aware of these factors when carrying out therapeutic interventions.

The finding of this study (Figure 8.5) suggests that both registered nurse (84%; *n* = 81) and student nurse (87%; *n* = 60) participants found this component of the ACCESS model useful or highly useful. It seems that mutual understanding between nurses and patients as a consequence of the application of the ACCESS model would foster a conducive relationship that would enhance a felt sense of value and recognition by patients (Ahuarangi, 1996; Narayanasamy, 1999).

According to Ahuarangi (1996), Peberdy (1997) and Narayanasamy (1999), the primary concern of nurses is to understand and deliver culturally sensitive care to diverse cultural groups. The finding confirms that many of the study participants found this aspect of the ACCESS model useful. Along with the rudiments of communication strategies identified in this model, nurses could embrace culturally adapted approaches to demonstrate sensitivity and considerations to patients' needs.

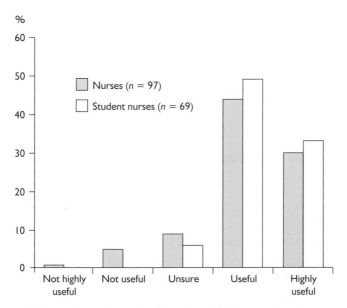

Figure 8.5 Delivering diverse culturally sensitive care to culturally diverse groups.

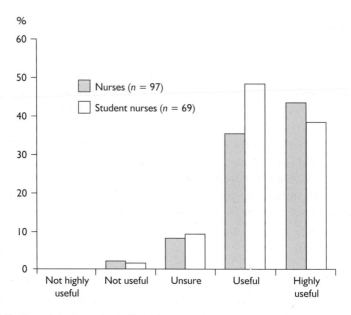

Figure 8.6 Fostering a culturally safe environment.

The findings with regard to the need for creation of cultural safety (Figure 8.6) suggest that many participants of this study found this aspect of the model useful or highly useful (registered nurses 95%; $n = 92$) (student nurses 90%; $n = 62$). Minority ethnic patients need to derive a sense of cultural safety (Ahuarangi, 1996; Polaschek, 1998). Patients who experience a sense of cultural safety are more likely to have trust in nurses and benefit further from the therapeutic relationship which is vital for interventions designed to meet cultural needs.

Limitations of the study

This study could have been followed up by interviews with participants to establish comparability between questionnaire responses and reflective accounts related to the usefulness of the ACCESS model. The model could have been piloted in other health care sites in the UK as part of case studies to establish its impact at a national scale. A further limitation of this study is that it did not seek users' perspectives about ACCESS as a model for transcultural care practice. User participation may offer further insights about its usefulness. However, plans are ahead to implement an evaluation study as part of action research, involving users and practitioners at various sites in the UK to establish the generalisability of the ACCESS model.

Conclusion

The overall findings of this study confirm that the ACCESS model offers a useful framework for nurses implementing transcultural care practice. The added value of the ACCESS model is that ACCESS as an acronym enables nurses to be consciously aware of its central features when carrying out nursing interventions in the care of minority ethnic patients. The conscious application of this model of transcultural nursing practice would enable nurses to internalise its component parts. It offers a comprehensive approach to transcultural nursing.

However, critics may point out that the ACCESS model is an oversimplification and that it is not explicit enough on the barriers to cultural care such as racism, power and oppression. These criticisms may be overcome if the issue of access to health care by minority ethnic groups is addressed as part of the ACCESS model.

The ACCESS model attempts to bring out the moral and ethical imperatives inherent in caring professionals. These include the motivation to be caring, compassionate and beneficial to those in health crisis and need. This model offers a moral and ethical premise for nurses to demonstrate the core values of nursing in the care of minority ethnic patients. The implication of this model is that it can be a useful guide for nurses attempting to provide culturally sensitive care for minority ethnic patients. Further studies are required to validate its usefulness in a variety of health care settings.

Acknowledgement

This chapter was published as an article in British Journal of Nursing, **11**(12), 643–50.

References

Ahmad, W. I. U. (1993) *Race and Health in Contemporary Britain*. Open University Press, Buckingham.

Ahuarangi, K. C. (1996) Creating a safe cultural space. *Kai Tiaki: Nursing New Zealand*, November, 13–15.

Altrichter, H., Posch, P. and Somekh, B. (1993) *Teachers Investigate their Work: An Introduction to the Methods of Action Research*. Routledge, London.

Baxter, C. (2000) Antiracist practice: achieving competency and maintaining professional standards. In: *Lyttle's Mental Health and Disorder* (eds. T. Thompson and P. Mathias), pp. 350–8. Baillière Tindall, Edinburgh.

Beishon, S., Virdee, S. and Hagell, A. (1995) *Nursing in a Multi-Ethnic NHS.* Policy Studies Institute, London.

Bhopal, R. (2001) Racism in medicine. The spectre must be exorcised. *British Medical Journal,* **322,** 1503–4.

Chady, S. (2001) The NSF for mental health from a transcultural perspective. *British Journal of Nursing,* **10**(15), 984–90.

Cohen, L. and Manion, L. (1989) *Research Methods in Education.* Routledge, London.

English National Board (2000) *Education in Focus, Strengthening Preregistration Nursing and Midwifery Education.* ENB, London.

Fernando, S. (1995) *Mental Health, Race and Culture.* Macmillan, London.

Gerrish, K. (1997) Preparation of nurses to meet the needs of an ethnically diverse society: educational implications. *Nurse Education Today,* **17,** 359–65.

Gerrish, K. and Papadopoulos, I. (1999) Transcultural competence: the challenge for nurse education. *British Journal of Nursing,* **8**(21), 1453–7.

Gerrish, K., Husband, C. and Mackenzie, J. (1996) *Nursing for a Multi-Ethnic Society.* University Press, Buckingham.

Goode, E. E. (1993) The cultures of illness. *US News and World Report,* **114**(6), 74–6.

Kleinman, A., Eisenberg, L. and Good, B. (1978) Culture, illness and care: clinical lessons. Anthropologic and cross-cultural research. *Annals of Internal Medicine,* **88,** 251–8.

Leininger, M. (1995) *Transcultural Nursing: Concepts, Theories and Practices.* McGraw-Hill, Berkshire.

Leininger, M. (1997) Transcultural nursing research to transcultural nursing education and practice. 40 years. *Image Journal of Nursing Scholarship,* **29**(4), 341–7.

Le Var, R. M. H. (1998) Improving educational preparation for transcultural health care. *Nurse Education Today,* **18,** 519–33.

McGee, P. (1993) *Issues in Transcultural Nursing: A Guide for Teachers of Nursing and Health.* Chapman & Hall, London.

McGee, P. (2000) Health, illness and culture. *Nursing Standard,* **14**(45), 33–4.

Middlesex University (2001) *Cultural Competence and Awareness Project.* Research Centre for Transcultural Studies in Health, Middlesex University.

Narayanasamy, A. (1998) *The ACCESS Model for Transcultural Mental Health Care.* University of Nottingham (unpublished).

Narayanasamy, A. (1999) Transcultural mental health nursing 2: race, ethnicity and culture. *British Journal of Nursing*, **8**(12), 741–4.

Papadopoulos, I. and Lees, I. (2002) Developing culturally competent research. *Journal of Advanced Nursing*, **37**(3), 258–63.

Papadopoulos, I., Tilki, M. and Taylor, G. (1998) *Transcultural Care: A Guide for Healthcare Professionals*. Quay, Wiltshire.

Peberdy, A. (1997) Communicating across cultural boundaries. In: *Debates and Dilemmas in Promoting Health: A Reader* (eds. M. Siddle, L. Jones, J. Katz and A. Peberdy), pp. 99–107. Open University, Buckinghamshire.

Polaschek, N. R. (1998) Cultural safety: a new concept in nursing people of different ethnicities. *Journal of Advanced Nursing*, **27**(3), 452–7.

Ramsden, I. (1993) Kawa Whakaruruhua: cultural safety in nursing education in Aotearoa (New Zealand). *Nursing Praxis*, **8**(3), 4–10.

Royal College of Nursing (1998) *The Nursing Care of Older People from Black and Minority Ethnic Communities*. Royal College of Nursing, London.

Rolfe, G., Freshwater, D. and Jasper, M. (2001) *Critical Reflection for Nurses*. Palgrave, Basingstoke.

Serrant Green, L. (2001) Transcultural nursing education: a view from within. *Nurse Education Today*, **21**(8), 670–8.

Stanley, S. (2000) Commentary: the cultural impact of Islam on the future direction of nurse education. *Nurse Education Today*, **20**(1), 69.

Sherer, J. L. (1993) Crossing cultures: hospitals begin breaking down the barriers to care. *Hospitals*, **67**(10), 29–31.

UKCC (1999) *Fitness for Practice. The UKCC Commission for Nursing and Midwifery Education*. UKCC, London.

Waterman, H., Tillen, D., Dickson, R. and de Koning, K. (2001) Action research: a systematic review and guidance for assessment. *Health Technology Assessment*, **5**(23), 1–166.

CHAPTER 9

Reflections and conclusion

Summary

This chapter reflects on central issues concerning my research and what factors motivated me to embark on a long and sustained investigation related to spiritual and cultural care. What follows is a summary of the various studies from the preceding chapters and their implications for nursing and nurse education, followed by recommendations. The final section examines the scope for further research.

Introduction

When I embarked on my research, I did not realise that it was going to be a long journey in my pursuit for empirical understanding of spiritual and cultural care. There was little literature or interest in spiritual or cultural care a decade or more ago. If spirituality was addressed in health, it was in the occasional paper by clerics or theologians or sources based on North American spirituality discourse. Modernism and its unquestioning faith in the scientific basis of medicine, sidelined spirituality to the realms of religious care or parapsychology, tainted as irrelevant in the contemporary industrial West. Spirituality was largely treated as a private and personal matter. At the time prevailing unwritten rules and values militated against those transgressing their roles as nurses and health carers when they attempted to address spiritual concerns. There were incidents where staff were warned not to dabble in spiritual matters and religious concerns, as these were considered to be the realms of the Chaplaincy. Equally, I witnessed several situations where minority groups' needs could have been dealt with more effectively, with respect for their dignity, showing greater compassion and care for their personhood. Anyone who did not fit the dominant values and norms of the prevailing health care culture was considered to be an outsider and a problem to be contained or referred to their families to meet their cultural and spiritual needs.

Some of the patients I looked after wanted to talk to me about their inner feelings and thoughts. These ranged from life and death matters, the meaning of life and suffering, conflicts and guilt and the need for forgiveness, their longing to be with friends and to be connected with their support network, their cultural needs and so on. The list concerning human inner suffering was endless. I felt inadequate and vulnerable when on numerous occasions in my clinical years I was ill equipped to deal with matters, largely inner ones affecting people's lives when they were facing illnesses. Sufferers felt empty, devastated, meaningless, desperate, estranged, confused, bewildered and disoriented. In a nutshell, the critical junctures in their lives, such as serious illness, had rendered them broken people. I was technically apt in dealing with needs that could be addressed by tangible measures. I was good at carrying out technical procedures and able to carry out conversations, but it remained superficial and confined to routine matters and social exchanges of niceties. When my conversation with patients veered towards matters that were central to their inner spirit, I steered away from these by using diversion techniques to focus on patients' physical problems. I drew from my knowledge of physiology and medicine, largely acquired uncritically from lecturers and book sources, to remain factual and objective when dealing with patients. I drew comfort from the fact that my medical knowledge provided me the shield to protect against my vulnerability when patients tried to share their inner and deeper issues affecting them. I was good at reading cardiograms and explaining about their intricacies to patients and staff. Many junior medical staff treated me as a vital resource, as they relied upon me to interpret cardiograms and predict second-degree heart block with great accuracy.

In spite of my technical qualities and professional knowledge I felt patients were missing something in their care. I was falling short in my role as a professional by unwittingly denying them holistic care, that is, care of the body, mind and spirit. This personal inadequacy led me to read the emerging literature on holistic care at that time, which reinforced my personal feeling of inadequacy with regard to holistic care in my professional capacity. These severe limitations led me to embark on a career as a researcher, teacher and practitioner of spirituality and culture. My first study (Narayanasamy, 1993) confirmed that nurses' knowledge and competence in spiritual care were impoverished due to inadequate educational preparation in spirituality.

All that was the past. I have moved on, but yet there is much more to do in promoting holistic approach to care. Remarkably, in the last two decades towards the end of the 20th century and the beginning of the 21st century, there has been a proliferation of literature, both conceptual and empirical papers and book sources in health care. Although postmodernism knocks all established disciplines of knowledge, including medicine, postmodern thinkers have actively encouraged and promoted the revival of interest in spirituality and cultural diversity. Consequently, New Age spirituality, New Religious Movements (NRMs), alternative medicine and complimentary therapies have proliferated, all offering a panacea for those disappointed in the failings of orthodox medicine and conventional science. One of the reasons for the rising popularity of complementary therapies is that they are person-centered and holistic in nature. Dr Deepak Chopra's books on body, mind and spirit are bestsellers because he attempts to bring a fusion of Western traditions and Eastern wisdom with regard to healing of the body and mind (Chopra, 1989). His holistic approach to healing resonates with the popular quest for spirituality that has been elusive due to modernism and its reliance on science and materialism. Although there have been great human achievements through science and materialism, these have failed to provide the fulfilment and contentment that individuals were looking for.

Spirituality is a durable term which has been with us since time immemorial. Early civilisation used it and perhaps truly understood it and used it holistically. Historical accounts of traditional health care illuminate the spiritual roots of nursing (Narayanasamy, 1999). One of the major problems that I constantly encountered in my early research is the lack of consensus about what constitutes spirituality. Ideas and discourses of spirituality abound in theology, philosophy and religious texts. Spirituality means many things to many people and it was often conflated with religion. Since the 1980s, beginning with the work of Simsen (1985), health care scholars in Britain have continued with the debate surrounding the concept of spirituality. Almost all writers converge on the perspective about the centrality of holistic care, that is, the care of the body, mind and spirit. The concept 'spirit' is seen as the essence of our being and one that gives us meaning and purpose in life. Its derivatives include a feeling of oneness, harmonious relationship with others and the environment, the need for forgiveness, relationship with a higher source, hope, trust and so on.

Spiritual care studies

From findings of the various studies in the book, it would appear that spiritual and cultural care are central to holistic care (see Table 9.1).

As given in Chapter 4, the study on chronic illness and spirituality illuminates that illness may become a spiritual encounter as well as a physical and emotional experience. Significantly, this study reveals that the lived experience of connectedness with God and others, and the search for meaning and purpose, appear to be important spiritual coping mechanisms during chronic illness. The experience of chronic illness may evoke a need in some patients to reach out to God in the belief and faith that help will be forthcoming to rescue them from

Table 9.1 Spiritual and cultural care studies.

Chapter	Studies	Page
4	Spiritual coping mechanisms in chronic illness	66
5	Critical incident study of nurses respond to the spiritual needs of their patients	85
6	Spirituality and learning disabilities: qualitative study	118
7	Transcultural nursing: how do nurses respond to cultural needs?	139
8	The ACCESS model: a transcultural nursing practice framework	159

their illness. Sometimes this intense need leads to the experience of a felt Divine Presence, which appears to be a spiritual resource that offers reassuring prospects of being helped through the crisis brought on by the illness. The patient's needs to be connected with God are established through prayers of petition, transaction and submission as spiritual coping mechanisms. A sense of hope, strength and security is derived from prayers.

The trajectory of chronic illness evokes a need for spiritual pursuits in terms of the search for meaning and purpose. This search is characterised by contemplation about the meaning of life with positive consequences such as a sense of peace and tranquillity. Aspects of coping strategies such as communicating with a Divine figure and feeling a Divine Presence are kept as private encounters with efforts to conceal them from others. This concealment is necessary for fear of being ridiculed if found out. When overt therapeutic support related to their spiritual need is not available patients continue to reflect a desire to be connected with other sources of support such as networks of families and friends. However, a point of consideration is that not all participants welcome spiritual resources of a religious nature.

The findings of this study are consistent with the results of other studies in which there is compelling evidence that patients resort to their spirituality and spiritual resources, including their faith, as coping mechanisms in chronic illness. It is clear that current evidence suggests that nurses and other health care practitioners need to be receptive and sensitive by being supportive to patients as they cope with their chronic illness.

Spiritual support for patients

An outline of the strategies derived from Narayanasamy (2005) is provided to assist nurses and other health care practitioners to enhance spiritual sup-

Table 9.2 Health care assessment of spiritual needs.

Obtaining detailed information about the patient's thoughts and feelings about the meaning and purpose of life, love and relationships, trust, hope and strength, forgiveness, expressions of beliefs and values.

Remaining sensitive to verbal and non-verbal cues from the patient.

Considerations about patient's abilities to see, hear and move are important factors that may later determine the relevance of certain interventions.

Observations of the ways in which the patient relates with people 'significant others' (people close to him, friends, and others who matter to him) may provide clues to the spiritual needs:

Does the patient welcome his visitors? Does their presence relax the patient or cause distress?

Does he get visitors from the church or religious community?

Observations of the patient's environment and significant objects/symbols related to his religious practice may give evidence of his spirituality.

port for patients. A spiritual history taking offers the practitioner the opportunity to understand their patients more holistically. Spiritual history as part of the assessment may provide insights into what gives meaning to individuals' lives. Assessment also opens up further insights into other important facets of patients' lives, which is at the root of compassionate care giving (Puchalski, 1999). Health care assessment of spiritual needs includes (see Table 9.2):

The other area of spiritual assessment includes attention to three factors: sense of meaning and purpose, means of forgiveness, and source of love and relationships. Observations and routine conversations with patients can lead to valuable information about each of these factors. Observations may include:

- How does the patient deal with other patients?
- Does he ruminate over past behaviours or how he has been treated by other people?
- How does the patient respond to criticism?

Spiritual support may include the considerations in Table 9.3.

If a member of the caring team feels unable to respond to a particular situation of spiritual need, then he or she should enlist the services of an appropriate individual. Health care interventions should be based on actions which reflect caring for the individual. There is no cure without caring. Caring signifies to the person that he or she is significant, and is worth someone taking the trouble to be concerned about them. Caring requires actions of support and assistance in growing. It means a non-judgmental approach and showing sensitivity to a

Table 9.3 Spiritual support.

- Respect for patients' spiritual and religious beliefs and practice.
- Acting as catalysts to help patients to access spiritual and religious advisers and facilities.
- Privacy and space for prayer/meditation.
- Facilitating attendance at religious services, prayer and worship meetings, listening to spiritual music and spiritual programmes on the radio or television, religious activities, maintaining specific religious customs.
- Welcoming visiting members and leaders of their spiritual community.
- Giving patients time and attention to talk about spiritual beliefs and concerns, especially about how these relate to their illness.
- Helping patients in their struggle and search for meaning and purpose in life.
- Aspects of support may include comfort, support, warmth, self-awareness, empathy, non-judgmental listening and understanding.

person's cultural values, physical preference and social needs. It demands an attitude of helping, sharing, nurturing and loving.

However, there is evidence in the literature that there is scope for improving the provisions for spiritual care. Although the NHS offers facilities such as departments for spiritual and pastoral services for meeting the spiritual needs of patients, nurses and other front line health care staff often act as companions to patients as they struggle with their illness. Sometimes the only source of hope and courage is spiritual resources for patients (Narayanasamy, 2004). The need for spiritual resources as coping mechanisms could be immediate, spontaneous and unpredictable. Nurses, as primary carers, have to respond to patients' needs in such situations and this means they would have to posses a working knowledge of how to respond to patients' spiritual needs as these emerge. There may not be the time for the organisation of planned and systematic care or time for calling members of the Department of Spirituality and Pastoral care to respond. Nurses have to respond to alleviate the spiritual distress before it escalates into an intractable problem.

When patients are experiencing crisis as a consequence of ill health they are likely to become spiritually distressed, and this state is probably indicative of the need for reassurance and comfort. According to Teasdale (1995), reassurance is an enduring process involving extensive interpersonal communication strategies that help to reduce patients' anxiety. However, participants appeared to have used the term 'comfort' to mean giving physical attention to make patients feel comfortable by being present by their bedside. In contrast,

Goldberg (1998) refers to this kind of intervention as 'presencing' and points out its benefits to patients. In developing a discourse on presencing derived from Roach (1991), Goldberg writes 'providing a presence which empowers and enables other to change, to accept, to grow, to die peacefully, is what nurses do each day' (p. 838). Moreover, in a phenomenological study of nurses' experiences, Dunniece and Slevin (2000, p. 614) suggest that 'presence' or 'being there' includes 'giving information, explaining, answering questions, listening and simply being present without speaking'. These authors provide evidence from their own study and others that the phenomenon of 'presence' or 'being there' is important in the care of cancer patients; however, they note that being there is more than a physical presence.

The ASSET model

The ASSET model (Actioning Spirituality and Spiritual care Education and Training in Nursing) is recommended as a possible option for improving spiritual care education in nursing. It should prove to be a useful framework and catalyst in effecting change in nurses' knowledge and understanding of the spiritual care requirements of patients. The essential components of this model are outlined in Table 9.4. Readers are advised to refer to Narayanasamy (1999) for further details of this model.

Although the ASSET model offers a workable framework for spiritual care interventions, it may appear to be too simplistic and trivial in its pursuit to explicate a complex phenomenon such as spirituality. Furthermore, a model depicting spirituality and spiritual care in such a narrow framework could be perceived to be consigning the spiritual dimension of humanity to a rigid regime in health care. However, a complex and sophisticated representation of spirituality and spiritual care interventions may render it an impossible task. As it is, health care is complex and the demands on health care professionals' time are huge, leaving little space for stretching an overcrowded programme of care aiming to meet the diverse needs of patients. There is elegance in simplicity and this is what the ASSET model aims to achieve. In this respect the ASSET model is flexible and could be easily accommodated and embedded in practice with perseverance. Nursing development units, in collaboration with staff of the spiritual and pastoral care departments, could use the ASSET model as a framework for instituting education and training programmes to promote spiritual care competence as an adjunct to other therapies among nurses and other health care professionals.

Chapters 5 and 6 comprise the findings of critical incident studies of nurses' responses to the spiritual needs of their patients, which have implica-

Table 9.4 The ASSET model (Narayanasamy, 2004).

Structure/content	Process	Outcome
Self awareness	Experiential learning related to value clarification: examination of personal values, prejudices, beliefs, assumptions and feelings	Value clarification; sensitivity and tolerance
Spirituality	Holism: care of the body, mind and spirit	Knowledgeable practitioner in spiritual dimensions of nursing.
	Perspectives of spirituality: classical and postmodern views, including New Age and eastern spiritualities	
	Broad aspects of spirituality – horizontal dimensions of spirituality, humanism and secularism	
Spiritual dimensions of nursing	Assessment: using spiritual assessment guide (see guide in Table 9.2)	Competence in assessment of spiritual care needs
	Planning and implementation: giving consideration to patients' individuality, privacy and space; listening and use of therapeutic self, the nurturing of the inner spirit; connection and presencing, comforting, compassion and unconditional love, being a companion in suffering, building trusting relationship	Planning spiritual needs-based care
		Being competent in counselling
		Positive nurse–patient relationship
		Competence in making judgement about effectiveness of spiritual dimensions of nursing
		Enhancing quality of care
		Spiritual integrity
		Healing and relief from spiritual pain
	Evaluation	

tions for nurse education and practice. Both studies are the first of their kind, offering scope for theory and practice development in nursing. In particular, these studies illuminate professional commitment to person-centredness, engagement, interpersonal attributes, involvement and sensitivity to cultural needs as features of ideal spiritual care practice (Tanyi, 2002; Sanders, 2002). However, the first critical incident study was limited in that the sample did not include learning disabilities nurses, so the study in Chapter 6 was developed to show how nurses caring for people with learning disabilities respond to clients' spiritual needs. This chapter addresses some of the gaps in the empirical work on learning disabilities in my earlier work (Narayanasamy, 1997).

Transcultural health care studies

Transcultural health care research maps out the extent of how nurses perceive and provide cultural care. Chapter 8 refers to a conceptual model and empirical data with regard to transcultural health care (see Table 8.1).

These chapters offer a model for transcultural nursing. It emerged in my work that spirituality and culture are integral to many peoples' lives. In particular, an apparent lack of transcultural perspectives on mental health care practice began to emerge. The ACCESS model is a unique and innovative development and is grounded in the theoretical perspectives derived from transcultural practice-based literature (Papadopoulos *et al.*, 1998; Peberdy, 1997; Leininger, 1997; Ahuarangi, 1996; Gerrish *et al.*, 1996; Goode, 1993; Sherer, 1993; Dobson, 1991) and empirical data derived from an unpublished survey study (Narayanasamy, 1998). The participants ($n = 36$) in this study who had educational input through this model suggest that 85% of respondents found it highly useful for transcultural mental health care practice.

The theoretical perspectives provided in Chapter 3 are influencing scholarly exposition on the subject of transcultural mental health care (Chady, 2001; Eisenbruch, 2001; Holland and Hogg, 2001). Chady developed a perspective on the 'NSF for mental health' that is based on this paper. This model formed the basis for the transcultural health care education offered at the University of Nottingham. The limitation of these papers is that it is based on a small sample and it is therefore difficult to generalise the application of the ACCESS model. However, according to Chady (2001, p. 988), 'the ACCESS model in its entirety creates a demand for training and supervision structures involving the experiences of culture-specific voluntary providers as well as the influence of expert panels'. An evaluation study of this model was reported in Chapter 8.

Chapter 8 provides empirical data from a study in which participants ($n = 166$) who received transcultural health care education completed questionnaires with statements about the usefulness of this model. The findings suggest that 90% ($n = 149$) of participants found the model to be very useful with respect to its various features. In spite of its limitations with respect to the lack of user perspectives on the usefulness of the model, this paper is valuable to the theory and practice of transcultural nursing and education. According to Chady (2001), Eisenbruch (2001), Holland and Hogg (2001) and Stanley (2000), the ACCESS model offers a useful framework for nurses implementing transcultural care practice. 'ACCESS' as an acronym enables nurses to be consciously aware of its central features when carrying out nursing care of minority ethnic patients. In summary, the ACCESS model is a unique development and there is empirical evidence from this publication to support its usefulness as a transcultural nursing framework.

Chapter 7 provides empirical data from a study of Registered Nurses ($n = 126$) to suggest that a majority of respondents claimed that they feel that patients' cultural needs should be given consideration. Cultural aspects of care seem to be a feature of the overall picture of nursing within the multicultural context of health care. Many participants claimed that they responded to the cultural needs of patients recently. A number of them felt that patients' cultural needs are adequately met, but these needs were perceived to be religious practices, diets, communication, dying, prayer and culture. Furthermore, a significant number of respondents suggested that they would like further education in meeting the cultural needs of their patients.

The main limitation of this study is that the relationship between nurses' experience and education could have been explored to establish the link between attitudes shaped by education and transcultural care practice. However, in spite of these limitations this study contributes to empirical understanding in nursing education and practice by offering insights into how nurses meet the cultural needs of their clients. The ACCESS model proposed in Narayanasamy (2002) guides curriculum developers in devising appropriate educational programmes for improving transcultural health care practices for nursing and nurse education.

The findings presented in this book make several original and independent contributions to knowledge. They integrate perspectives drawn from a variety of sources, including empirical data derived from personal and collaborative studies of spirituality and culture. The theories and practice of spiritual and cultural care developed through this research programme are being used by three branches of nursing (adult, mental health and learning disabilities) and pastoral care nationally and internationally.

The two models, ACCESS and ASSET, are unique and innovative developments offering frameworks for cultural care practice and spiritual care education and training respectively (Clegg, 2003; Chady, 2001; Eisenbruch, 2001; Holland and Hogg, 2001; Stanley, 2000; Tanyi, 2001; McSherry, 2000). The critical incident technique studies (Chapters 5 and 6) are unique methodologically and offer data theories on how nurses provide spiritual care. The qualitative study (Chapter 4) advances the theory that the trajectory of chronic illness involves a spiritual coping mechanism where connectedness with God through prayer and connectedness with others appear to be significant as part of the healing process. This research programme uniquely offers a model for a sustained and coherent approach to the development of spiritual and cultural care knowledge and practice.

Limitations

Many of the limitations of the various studies were addressed in earlier chapters. A further limitation of this project is that it addresses a diverse range of studies on spirituality and culture and may appear fragmented. However, attempts were made to minimise this by reflecting the developmental nature of the project, with further research studies designed to advance knowledge and practice. Gaps in the early theoretical literature were addressed in subsequent work. The multi-perspectives and methodologies offered method and theoretical triangulation in the generation of rich qualitative data and subsequent theory development. Much of the data generation depended upon qualitative research techniques, but this was not due to an aversion to positivism, but became imperative because of the holistic and multi-perspective nature of spiritual and cultural care experiences. A positivist approach, using probability sampling with methods designed to control variables, may not lend itself to the generation of rich data from the lived experiences of participants.

The findings of the various studies in this book add to the existing body of knowledge. The research is unique, original and pioneering. Many aspects of the spiritual and cultural research are in line with the theory and research presented by other writers, but at the same time, make an original contribution to the understanding and practice of spiritual and cultural care. The theoretical insights derived from my research were subsequently published in a variety of sources (see Narayanasamy, 2001) and continue to guide many students, nurse teachers and practitioners (Hawley, 2002). Contemporary scholars demonstrate the influence of the research in this book in guiding their discourses on spirituality (Aveyard, 1995; McSherry, 2000; Fry, 1997; Ross, 1997; Govier, 2000; Swinton, 2001; Thorpe and Barsely, 2001; Pesut, 2002; Tanyi, 2002; Sanders, 2002) and culture (Clegg, 2003; Chady, 2001; Eisenbruch, 2001; Holland and Hogg, 2001; Stanley, 2000). A web site has been set up in response to the increasing national and international interest in the spiritual and cultural research presented in this book (Bearings Project, 2002).

Reflexive account: a spiritual journey

As I was putting the finishing touches to the book, I went back to my reflective notes that I maintained throughout my research. I have extracted some bits of material from these notes to provide reflexive accounts of spiritual encounters in my journey as a researcher. Soon after the interviews or contacts with research participants, I reflected on my encounters and interaction with participants and recorded these experiences. According to Smith (1996), cited in Swinton (2001), the researcher serves as the primary instrument through which data are collected. A reflective journal can help researchers to gather evidence of their continuing engagement with participants as well as revelations of the self as the researcher enters into the stages of the research process (Swinton, 2001).

According to Johns (1998), a careful recording of the dialogue that takes place between a researcher and participant guides reflection. It enables the researcher to look back and analyse the patterns of reflection. I used elements of the Model of Structured Reflection (MER) to guide my reflection (see Johns, 1998). Johns (1998) suggests that through reflections, practitioners can begin to gain understanding of ways of knowing in terms of ethics, empirical evidence and so on.

As I reflected upon the interviews that I had conducted as part of the qualitative studies of spiritual care, including the study identified in Chapter 4, several themes emerged. These are typified as spiritual encounters, spiritual healing, mistaken identity, impression management, participants as co-researchers, unintended outcomes and transformation.

Spiritual encounter

The interviews became a spiritual encounter as well as a data-gathering process. During the interviews I was gaining access to the personal and private world of the participants. As the relationship, albeit a transient one, became a trust-building process, the participants began to open up their private world with regard to the lived experience of their spirituality. Montgomery (1991) refers to such a relationship as a spiritual transcendence. By this, Montgomery means that there is connectedness between two people – the experience becomes a spiritual journey leading to spiritual growth and development. The interviewer engages the participants in reflections and interpretation about their lived experience. According to Taylor (1998), reflection is central to making sense of human existence, as lived experiences provide the impetus to accumulate and gather interpretative significance when events are remembered. By reflecting about what has happened and is happening to themselves, to others and to other things of significance, people generally develop an awareness of meaning relevant to themselves and others. In an edited book, Johns and Freshwater (1998) suggest that reflections ultimately lead to transformation. As a researcher, transformation inevitably takes place in myself as I reflect during the interaction and the discourse that emerges at interviews. Further reflections take place as I analyse the data. In a way, data interpretation leads to transformation in that new insights are gained. I became transformed as a consequence of the new insights. The participants became transformed as a result of the interactions between the researcher and themselves.

Trust in the researcher leads to a sense of safety and security. I suggest elsewhere (see Narayanasamy, 2002) that in cultural negotiations a sense of trust and safety is necessary. Likewise, McSherry (2000) postulates that the need for a trusting relationship is part of our spirituality. This author recounts incidents in which trusting relationships and environments appear to be significant in meeting the patients' spiritual needs. The interactions in interview situations develop and progress as a sense of trust is felt. This sense of trust, security and safety helped me to enter the private world of the participants in my research, as mentioned earlier.

In spite of the positive aspects of the spiritual encounters in interviews, there is a downside to encounters of such a nature. The relationship is a transient one and the positive relationship and connectedness has to come to an end. I found that as an interviewer I had to 'let go' and terminate the interview. Likewise, the participants had to do the same. In some situations it had been hard for both of us, but such encounters had to come to an end for apparent reasons. Agreeing with participants about a clear agenda and time limit for the interview before it starts may help departures to be less painful or avoid disappointments. I found a short debriefing session at the end of the interview helped to 'let go' the relationship that was established within the brief encounter.

What follows is a reflective account of some spiritual encounters. This incident concerns a participant who was awaiting test results. Jim, a medical patient, appeared angry as I approached him for the interview. He intimated to me that he was totally 'unhappy about being dumped' into a side room following his transfer from another hospital. At this point I recalled what the nurse had said about this patient when I approach her before starting the interview. Jim had to be nursed in a side room because he had been exposed to a potential risk of developing a serious cross-infection following a major heart surgery in a hospital at another district. He was transferred to this hospital and as a precautionary measure, while awaiting confirmation of the laboratory report, it was decided that he should be nursed in a side room according to the hospital policy. Jim appeared to be unaware of this. He also implied that he had not received his prescribed medication since his admission. I told Jim that I would get the nurse to explain his treatment and proceeded to fetch the nurse. The nurse told me that she would be happy for me to offer any explanation the patient wish to seek.

I went back to the side room and informed Jim that I would be more than happy to discuss his concerns. I listened, giving Jim adequate time to ventilate his anger and feelings and showed genuine concern for what he had to say. Jim demanded that he wanted to see the doctor. I replied that this can be arranged and he then began to calm down. I asked the named nurse to contact the doctor in order to comply with the patient's request. I offered to be present when the doctor came to see Jim and to clarify anything that the doctor said. Jim began to feel more relaxed when he realised that something positive was actually happening. On seeing some results, Jim asked me if I was the charge nurse, although I indicated earlier that I was a researcher and had arranged to interview him. Jim also hinted that he wished that I was present when he was admitted and he felt that the misunderstanding could have been avoided. I clarified again about my status as a researcher. I felt good that I had done something that brought some comfort to the patient. My earlier findings (see Narayanasamy and Owen, 2001) on critical incidents of spiritual care suggest that nurses derive greater satisfaction when they provide spiritual care. Following this small gesture on my part, the interview proceeded.

However, soon after the interview I reflected on the above incident and several strands of spirituality emerged in my head. Jim's state of mind and anger were probably indications that he was seeking the opportunity to:

- Ventilate his anger and feelings
- Communicate with someone about his anxieties and fears
- Receive compassion and care

On my part, elements of spirituality may also be traced in my intuitive responses to Jim's needs as follows:

- Being caring and showing compassion which featured as giving time and attention, and showing genuine concern
- Taking practical action in response to his need to see the doctor
- My presence (having calming effect)

The effects of my intervention upon this patient were that he felt calm and relaxed and expressed his gratitude to me for being caring and showing compassion. In return, this encounter gave me a sense of fulfilment, i.e. my intervention brought about a positive and beneficial outcome. In other words, the spiritual nature of my encounter with this patient was that it gave me a sense of meaning and purpose as a direct result of my intervention, albeit in an *ad hoc* and unplanned way. This incident raises the question of how many times nurses and other health carers undertake activities of this nature that are uncharted as spiritual care interventions. It is clear that nursing can be a service to human kind, requiring commitment to some others. Serving others takes on a deeper dimension of loving and caring as one promotes wellness. This involves the process in which spiritual resources of the nurse are shared with others (Narayanasamy, 1999; Montgomery, 1991; Jacik, 1986).

Another interview with a participant became a spiritual encounter as well. Jack, a research participant, felt uplifted and inspirational towards the end of the interview, although I was clear in my head that there were no overt gestures of spiritual care on my part. At the end of the interview Jack asked if he could pray with me. I obliged and he prayed both in words and contemplatively. As he prayed, within moments I felt a unique sensation: I felt peaceful and unexplainably happy. Something descended upon us which was beyond comprehension, and I am sure that it must have been something spiritual that defies words or description. I thanked Jack for his prayers. Perhaps there is something therapeutic about prayers which benefits researchers as well!

Spiritual healing

In a research of this nature, the researcher may become a 'shoulder to cry' on. Several participants became emotional and tearful as they told me their stories about their lived experience. In some interviews I became a counsellor, comforter, supporter and companion. I shared with the participants their emotions, happiness, pain, anguish and so on as they relived their experiences of happier occasions, as well as traumatic and painful events. But nevertheless, participants were willing to pour out their pent-up emotions. They needed no prompts, but time with an interested person who was willing to listen unconditionally and non-judgmentally about their experience. I recall that two participants used the interview as therapeutic situations to move through personal crises as consequences of bereavement. One participant was extremely emotional, filled with a great sense of guilt feelings about the death of a loved one. There were unfinished business, self-blame and sadness about the untimely death of his partner. This incident posed an ethical dilemma for me as a researcher. This reaction emerged in the middle of the interview. My reflections-in-practice were: should I tactfully terminate the interview and refer the participant to the official counsellor, or act as a companion to offer support at that moment of crisis? Aldridge (2000) suggests that in such moments of crises or critical junctures in people's lives, spiritual support and resources may be helpful and therapeutic. My inner voice – maybe intuition was called into play – told me to support the participant. I listened, comforted and supported the participant. I remained as the participant's companion during his recollections about the traumatic experience and anguish. I became the 'shoulder to cry' on and the participant continued to share inner thoughts and feelings. As a consequence of my therapeutic approach the participant became calmer and peaceful following the release of pent-up emotions that this individual had been carrying for so long. This participant thanked me for being understanding, supporting and comforting. As I reflect, this cameo is a reminder of a broken person who has been in spiritual crisis for some time. Jacik (1986) identifies the spiritual nature of nursing in which carers become a companion to another's journey, not a problem solver or a rescuer, just a companion. This entails serious reflection about the concerns of another, being present when needs arise and sensing one's own helplessness and brokenness in that of another.

Spiritual support can be ad hoc and unplanned

The above encounter was a spiritual one for both of us. The research participant derived peace and possibly forgiveness as a result of our encounter. As a researcher it was a privilege to be allowed access to the inner turmoil of the participant. This reminded me that a positivist approach using probability sampling, controls and measurable tools may not have been as revealing about the lived experience of participants. Reflecting on practice, I have unknowingly provided spiritual support for the participant. I listened and gave unconditional time and attention. I comforted and supported a fellow human in crisis. It is a reminder that spiritual crisis can occur at anytime and *ad hoc* spiritual care and support may be required to help distressed individuals. My willingness to be a companion during this crisis provided the catharsis and probably started the spiritual healing that this individual has been longing for. In a way, I had been a spiritual healer, although my primary task was to interview the participant as a researcher. Both the participant and I have spiritually grown and developed, and perhaps transformed as a consequence of the experience and encounter. Transformation took place in the sense that I learnt from this experience and I am able to share such experience with readers.

As I reflected on practice as a researcher I recalled another incident. Another research participant, David, was full of anger and bitterness as a result of the dreaded diagnosis 'Cancer'. At the beginning of the interview David, a believer and a Methodist, was bitter and angry towards God and the impotence of the medical profession with regard to his ailment. David's response was

... why me? why now?, when I have led a clean and pious way of life so far, when Jack who lives across the road where I live has led a careless and carefree live full of vices is healthy.

David's anger was directed towards his God for letting him down so badly, when as a devout Christian he had led an unblemished and virtuous life, resisting temptations and vices. Understandably, he was full of blame about the ineffectiveness of the health service to provide a cure for his condition. David felt let down by the system and expressed that more could be done to rid him of his cancer. David appeared to have bottled up all of these catastrophic events until our encounter at the interview. Again as a researcher, I faced an ethical dilemma like the preceding one about the best course of action to follow. My intuitive response was to listen and support David, so I did exactly that. Scholars such as Moore (1903), Pritchard (1912) and Ross (1939) have developed a discourse about the role of intuition in ethical decisions making. These scholars argue that sometimes we have to let our inner moral faculty (intuition) guide us when we face ethical challenges. In other words, our inner voice tells us what is the right thing to do intuitively. According to Ross (1939), when we are faced with an ethical dilemma or conflicting duties, the right thing to do is to fulfil our duties. With regard to my ethical dilemma, I felt guided by my inner voice (intuition). The right thing to do was to support the participant during his crises.

The participant became calmer after he had the opportunity to vent his pent-up emotions and feelings related to the catastrophic news that was going to change and shorten his life. On reflection, it appears as though I have been a useful companion in the participant's journey at this critical juncture in his life. The news of the diagnosis was a critical juncture; it became a spiritual encounter, posing challenges to the meaning and purpose of his life. I had to fill the gap that the consultant had left and help the participant to move on. I have been a spiritual facilitator, enabling the participant to make sense of the chaos and bewilderment as a consequence of the news of the diagnosis.

Mistaken identity

Some participants in the research mistook my identity and assumed that I was a doctor. Others took me for a priest or counsellor or psychologist. I felt honoured but false in the light of the mistaken identities. I had to correct the misinterpretation, but felt that perhaps I was too professional or perhaps appeared too boring. However, once the record was straightened the interviews proceeded reasonably well. When certain participants realised that I wanted to talk about things to do with their spirituality, for example, one of them expressed 'Am I on my last legs?'. I had to reassure the participant that this was not the case. The other incident of mistaken identity was concerning the patient in a side room, a subject which I have already covered above.

Participants as co-researchers

Participants were co-researchers, as their partnership and cooperation with this enterprise helped the research to be materialised. They owned the data and were major stakeholders. They had the keys to the source of knowledge and understanding. I was the medium and conveyor of their message. I became the technician who pieced together their stories. As co-researchers they were active partners in providing and validating the stories about their lived experience. They ensured that the research was valid ecologically by being reality checkers. My gratitude to them is profound as their influence upon my personal growth and development has been great.

Impression management

As a researcher I had to work hard at impression management. I had to portray the image of a professional by following an appropriate dress code, etiquette and mannerism. I had to uphold trustworthiness and gain the confidence of participants. I made efforts to be an enabler and facilitator with effective communication skills as an interviewer. I had to enter the private world of participants. I ensured that I 'bracketed out' my own thoughts, perspectives etc. and adopted measures such as avoidance of misleading questions to minimise bias. I followed strict ethical guidelines and protocols and treated the privilege of access to participants' private and personal worlds with great respect, sensitivity and care. The trust bestowed upon me had to be upheld and safeguarded. The whole process of impression management had to be displayed to participants, research fund providers, colleagues and others connected to the research project. My integrity and credibility had to be maintained. Finally, I had to ensure that my trustworthiness as custodian of the data provided by participants was beyond reproach.

Unintended outcomes of research work

As I reflected about my approach in interviews with participants it appears that I had unwittingly used the Rogerian counselling techniques (Rogers, 1991). I had given participants attention, time and unconditional positive regard. Non-judgmentally I listened to their stories and accepted them. I was interested in what they had to say. I was supportive, comforting and encouraging, without asking misleading questions or being over enthusiastic to miss out vital information. There appeared to be positive relationship between participants and myself. In most instances we connected and there were incidents where my therapeutic interventions were active, although *ad hoc*, and I had to make ethical decisions as whether to go beyond my remit as a researcher. Interviews can be testing, as unpredictable things may happen, and researchers have to think on their feet, improvise and react to alleviate problems or help participants when they become distressed as we unwittingly touch their inner core, their spirit. Interviews involving explorations of experiences, feelings, emotions and reflections may result in highly charged reactions and vulnerability. My intuitive response was to intervene in desperate situations, as discussed earlier. Leaving a distressed individual is inhumane and potentially damaging, and my interventions have always attempted to bring about positive outcomes.

Transformation

As hinted earlier in my discussion, transformation was multilateral, as it took place in participants and myself. There were personal growth and development in both parties. I gained new insights about the phenomenon of spirituality and illness/crises. The experience has been a spiritual encounter and ethically challenging, and *ad hoc* measures were instituted to help individuals in crisis. We connected in the process of our transient encounters, but soon departed when the transaction came to end. Participants, and perhaps myself, experienced spiritual healing. Unwittingly I was drawn into spiritual care – I became a spiritual facilitator and healer. As I reflected on my role as a researcher/field worker, I became a changed person – a transformation had taken place – the most important process of reflections.

My journey as a practitioner, researcher and teacher has been a challenging one and one that has involved many trials and errors. There were so many examples, such as trying to gain the trust of research participants, trying to break the barriers to spiritual care, and trying to put in place a compassionate presence, including finding a common language so that both of us could carry out our transactions pertaining to spirituality by avoiding dialogues in which ambiguities and professional imperialism might intervene unwittingly on my part. I constantly had to remind myself that I had to remain consciously aware of my need to be at ease in the unnatural setting of an interview at times, ensuring bracketing, empathy and humility. Constantly I had to prevent myself from transgressing the boundaries of empathy and humility due to overzealousness in my pursuit of data. Almost all interviews involved a great degree of emotional labour as I entered into a relationship with participant, though a transient one, as part of the research process that taps into the lived experience of patients as they cope with chronic illness. Sociologists have identified the taxing nature of work involving emotional labour, which can be draining and exhausting (Hochschild, 1983). In contrast, in spite of the emotional labour involved in interviews of this nature, my experiences have largely been positive and mutually beneficial.

Conclusion

Writing this book has been a challenge, in that a range of studies had to be pieced together to make a coherent presentation of many years of research work and endurance to make sense of complex and diverse topics of care such as spirituality and culture. I have charted a series of conceptual and empirical studies and their findings as well as trajectories of experiences involving participants and myself as a researcher. The reflexive accounts provided me with an opportunity to share some of the unintended outcomes of studies. I guess these were inevitable as we enter and perhaps intrude, albeit unwittingly, into other people's private worlds. It has been a privilege to be allowed access for data gathering. A wealth of data has become available through the cooperation of participants, who were willing to set aside time for my research investigations. I am gratefully indebted to them all.

The research programme presented in this book has led to the development of the ASSET and ACCESS models, which will continue to make an impact upon spiritual and cultural care practice and education. In this respect the research makes a major contribution to the theory and practice of spiritual and cultural care in nurse education and practice. Finally, the conceptual and empirical work presented in this book provide a body of evidence which can guide curriculum and practice developments related to spiritual and cultural dimensions of care.

References

Ahuarangi, K. C. (1996) Creating a safe cultural space. *Kai Tiaki: Nursing New Zealand*, November, 13–15.

Aldridge, D. (2000) *Spirituality, Healing and Medicine*. Jessica Kingsley, London.

Aveyard, B. (1995) A question of faith. *Nursing Standard*, **9**(37), 45–6.

Bearings Project, The (2002) http://www.nottingham.ac.uk/healthquest/staff/an-bearingsproject.html.

Chady, S. (2001) The NSF for mental health from a transcultural perspective. *British Journal of Nursing*, **10**(15), 984–90.

Chopra, D. (1989) *Quantum Healing; Exploring the Frontiers of Mind/body Medicine*. Bantam, New York.

Clegg, A. (2003) Older South Asian patient and carer perceptions of culturally sensitive care in a community hospital setting. *Journal of Clinical Nursing*, **12**, 283–90.

Dobson, S. (1991) *Transcultural Nursing: A Contemporary Imperative*. Scutari, London.

Dunniece, U. and Slevin, E. (2000) Nurses' experience of being present with a patient receiving a diagnosis of cancer. *Journal of Advanced Nursing*, **32**(3), 611–18.

Eisenbruch, M. (2001) *National Review of Nursing Education: Multicultural Nursing Education*. Department of Education, Training and Youth Affairs, Commonwealth of Australia.

Fry, E. (1997) Spirituality: connectedness through being and doing. In: *Spirituality: The Heart of Nursing* (ed. S. Ronaldson). Alismed Publications, Melbourne.

Gerrish, K., Husband, C. and Mackenzie, J. (1996) *Nursing for a Multiethnic Society*. University Press, London.

Goldberg, B. (1998). Connection: an exploration of spirituality in nursing care. *Journal of Advanced Nursing*, **27**, 836–42.

Goode, E. E. (1993) The cultures of illness. *US News and World Report*, **114**(6), 74–6.

Govier, I. (2000) Spiritual care in nursing: a systematic approach. *Nursing Standard*, **14**(17), 32–6.

Hawley, G. (2002) Book review: Spiritual care. *Nurse Education Today*, **22**(8), 669.

Holland, K. and Hogg, C. (2001) *Cultural Awareness in Nursing and Health Care: An Introductory Text*. Arnold, London.

Hochschild, A. R. (1983) *The Managed Heart: Commercialization of Human Feeling*. University of California Press, Berkeley.

Jacik, M. (1986) Personal communcation. In: *Spiritual Dimensions of Nursing Practice* (ed. V. B. Carson). W. B. Saunders Company, Philadelphia.

Johns, C. (1998) Opening the doors of perception. In *Transforming Nursing Through Reflective Practice* (eds. C. Johns and D. Freshwater), pp. 1–28. Blackwell Science, Oxford.

Johns, C. and Freshwater, D. (1998) *Transforming Nursing Through Reflective Practice*. Blackwell Science, Oxford.

Leininger, M. (1997) Transcultural nursing research to transcultural nursing education and practice. 40 years. *Image Journal of Nursing Scholarship*, **29**(4), 341–7.

McSherry, W. (2000) *Making Sense of Spirituality in Nursing Practice*. Churchill Livingstone, Edinburgh.

Montgomery, C. (1991) The care-giving relationships: paradoxical and transcendent aspects. *Journal of Transpersonal Psychology*, **23**, 91–105.

Moore, G. E. (1903) *Principia Ethica*. Cambridge University Press, Cambridge.

Narayanasamy, A. (1993) Nurses awareness and preparedness in meeting their patients spiritual needs. *Nurse Education Today*, **13**(4), 196–201.

Narayanasamy, A. (1997) Spiritual dimensions of learning disability. In *Dimensions of Learning Disabilities* (eds. B. Gates and C. Beacock). Baillière Tindall, London.

Narayanasamy, A. (1998) *The ACCESS Model for Transcultural Mental Health Care*. University of Nottingham (unpublished).

Narayanasamy, A. (1999) Learning spiritual dimensions of care from a historical perspective. *Nurse Education Today*, **19**, 386–95.

Narayanasamy, A. (2001) *Spiritual Care: A Practical Guide for Nurses and Health Care Practitioners*, 2nd edn. Wiltshire, Quay.

Narayanasamy, A. (2002) The ACCESS model: a transcultural nursing practice framework. *British Journal of Nursing*, **11**(9), 643–50.

Narayanasamy, A. (2004) The puzzle of spirituality. *British Journal of Nursing*, **13**(19), 1141–4.

Narayansamy, A. (2005) *Psychological and spiritual support.* In: *Supportive Care for the Urology Patient* (eds. R. W. Norman and D. C. Currow), pp. 55–76. Oxford University Press, Oxford.

Narayanasamy, A. and Owens, J. (2001) A critical incident study of nurses' responses to the spiritual needs of their patients. *Journal of Advanced Nursing*, **33**(4), 446–55.

Papadapoulos, I., Tilki, M. and Taylor, G. (1998) *Transcultural Care: A Guide for Healthcare Professionals.* Quay Books, Wiltshire.

Peberdy, A. (1997) Communicating across cultural boundaries. In: *Debates and Dilemmas in Promoting Health: A Reader* (eds. M. Siddle, L. Jones, J. Katz and A. Peberdy), pp. 99–107. Open University, Buckinghamshire.

Pesut, B. (2002) The development of nursing students' spirituality and spiritual care-giving. *Nurse Education Today*, **22**, 128–35.

Puchalski, C. M. (1999) Taking a spiritual history: FICA. *Spirituality Medicine. Connect*, **3**, 1.

Pritchard, H. A. (1912) Does moral philosophy rest on a mistake? *Mind*, **21**, 21–37; reprinted in *Moral Obligation: Essays and Lectures.* Clarendon Press, Oxford.

Roach, M. (1991) The call to consciousness: compassion in today's health world. In: *In Caring: The Compassionate Healer* (eds. L. Gaul and M. Leininger), pp. 7–18. National League for Nursing. New York.

Rogers, C. (1991) *On Becoming a Person.* Constable, London.

Ross, W. D. (1939) *The Foundations of Ethics.* Oxford University Press, Oxford.

Ross, L. (1997) *Nurses' Perceptions of Spiritual Care. Developments in Nursing and Health Care.* Avebury, Aldershot.

Sanders, C. (2002) Challenge for spiritual care-giving in the millennium. *Contemporary Nurse*, **12**(2), 107–11.

Sherer, J. L. (1993) Crossing cultures: hospitals begins breaking down the barriers to care. *Hospitals*, **67**(10), 29–31.

Simsen, B. (1985) Spiritual needs and resources in illness and hospitalisation. *Unpublished Masters Thesis.* University of Manchester.

Smith, B. A. (1996) The problem drinker's lived experience of suffering: a hermeneutic phenomenological study. *Unpublished MSc Nursing Thesis.* University of Aberdeen. Cited in Swinton, J. (2001) *Spirituality and Mental Health Care.* Jessica Kingsley, London.

Stanley, S. (2000) Commentary: the cultural impact of Islam on the future of direction of nurse education. *Nurse Education Today*, **20**(1), 69.

Swinton, J. (2001) *Spirituality and Mental Health Care*. Jessica Kingsley, London.

Swinton, J. (2002) *A Space to Listen: Meeting the Spiritual Needs of People with Learning Disabilities*. The Foundation for People with Learning Disabilities, London.

Tanyi, R. A. (2002) Towards clarification of the meaning of spirituality. *Journal of Advanced Nursing*, **39**(5), 500–9.

Taylor, B. (1998) Locating a phenomenological perspective of reflective nursing and midwifery practice by contrasting interpretative and critical reflection. In: *Transforming Nursing through Reflective Practice* (eds. C. Johns and D. Freshwater). Blackwell Science, Oxford.

Teasdale, K. (1995) Theoretical and practice considerations on the use of reassurance in the nursing management of anxious patients. *Journal of Advanced Nursing*, **22**(1), 79–86.

Thorpe, K. and Barsley, J. (2001) Healing through reflection. *Journal of Advanced Nursing*, **35**(5), 760–8.

Index